HIV and culture confluence:
Cross-cultural experiences on HIV, gender and education from Johannesburg conference

HIV and culture confluence: Cross-cultural experiences on HIV, gender and education from Johannesburg conference

Table of contents

7   About this book
9   Foreword
11 Acronyms

13 HIV and culture confluence - 'Changing the River's Flow': Possibilities and challenges in programming
    (Lois Chingandu, Ngoni Chibukire and Maserame Mojapele)

25 SAfAIDS Changing the River's Flow Model: A social ecological behaviour change intervention for HIV prevention in southern Africa
    (Lois Chingandu, Ngoni Chibukire and Maserame Mojapele)

37 The Innovation Fund: Supporting education, gender and HIV prevention
    (Olloriak Sawade and Jeanette Kloosterman)

51 Communicating HIV and AIDS, sexuality and gender messages across cultures: The place of a newsletter in an Internet era
    (Eliezer F. Wangulu)

63 Sexual and reproductive desires and practices of Kenyan young positives: Opportunities for skills building through social media
    (Anke van der Kwaak, Francis Obare and Hermen Ormel)

71 Monitoring and Evaluation: Measuring for change (Jan Reynders)

87 About the authors

About this book

In April 2010, Southern Africa HIV/AIDS Information Dissemination Service (SAfAIDS), the Dutch affiliate of the international Oxfam organisation (Oxfam Novib), the Humanist Institute for Development Cooperation (Hivos) and the Royal Tropical Institute (KIT) organised a forum to share experiences on implementing interventions to address HIV and AIDS, sexuality, gender and education. Culture was a cross-cutting issue at the conference.

The Cross-cultural Learning Conference (CCLC) was held in Johannesburg, South Africa, and brought together regional, national and community groups from Africa, Asia, Europe, the Middle East and Latin America. The conference sought to provide a platform for sharing good practices and examining the role of culture in HIV and AIDS prevention and mitigation among participants working in training, home-based care, education, advocacy, lobbying and information production and dissemination, among others.

The participants, who included traditional leaders, researchers, community workers, programme implementers, government representatives, development agencies, policy makers, NGO representatives, media and donors, hoped that at the end of the meeting, they would be equipped with knowledge, skills and tools for sharing within their organisations in order to improve their work.

A number of information products have been developed from the conference to facilitate wider sharing of the event's outcomes. KIT dedicated the June 2010 edition of *Exchange on HIV and AIDS, Sexuality and Gender* quarterly magazine and its Portuguese version, *Intercambio,* to the conference outcomes. Also, a conference report compiled by SAfAIDS was shared among partners, participants and stakeholders and a documentary on the conference produced. This book and its French version are some of the avenues through which key conference outcomes are being shared.

This book targets professionals involved in an array of projects or programmes in the areas of HIV and AIDS, sexual and reproductive health, gender and education mainly working with NGOs, faith-based organisatiions (FBOs) and community-based organisations (CBOs). It is also aimed at policy makers and programme managers in governmental institutions, international NGOs (INGOs), UN agencies, media personnel, researchers and teachers. The objective of the book is to empower these target readers with skills to improve the way they implement their programmes.

Eliezer F. Wangulu
Editor
Royal Tropical Institute
Amsterdam, The Netherlands

Foreword

Decades of experience and research demonstrate that seeking to influence behaviour alone is insufficient and unsustainable if the underlying factors that influence behaviours such as poverty and culture are not also considered. In 1999 UNAIDS identified culture as one of the five leading domains responsible for worsening the HIV epidemic alongside spirituality, gender, social and economic factors.

Culture is a creation of human beings who have attached a lot of meaning to it. Humans are suspended in webs of significance they themselves have spun. A failure of modernity has been the inability to grasp how people weave meaning from those webs to determine their behaviours.

It is therefore gratifying to note that the Cross-cultural Learning Conference, which I personally attended and which was jointly organised by SAfAIDS, Oxfam Novib, Hivos and KIT, placed culture at the centre of all the deliberations by participants at the South Africa event. The conference provided a forum through which delegates learned not only about the diverse socio-historical and cultural contexts within which HIV thrives, but also about the influence of culture, gender-based violence (GBV) and the role of education in combating them.

Therefore programmes addressing these issues should be locally-driven and culturally-appropriate. Although culture and HIV are highlighted in statistics, organisations have not significantly or systematically shaped their strategies and work around culture. We applaud SAfAIDS for taking an initiative in looking at empirical evidence, to tackle the triple linkage on gender, culture and HIV through innovative community-driven interventions in southern Africa.

A major lesson from the conference was that if we want to change harmful cultural practices, we should not adopt a top-down approach. There is a need for dialogue within communities and the recognition and identification of cultural practices that violate human rights or/and result in the spread of HIV. It is through individual and community dialogue that change can be realised.

I would like to turn briefly to two key recommendations reached at the conference. One of them reminded us of the value of culture in HIV and gender programmes by imploring us to recognise the capacity of communities to address negative cultural practices. We should, as practitioners, encourage positive/protective cultural practices and discourage negative ones which drive HIV transmission and/or promote gender inequality. Secondly, education plays a key role in reaching our aims and goals. Therefore education must be offered by various stakeholders and through various approaches such as schools, medical services, family, media and peers to reinforce the message of gender, education and HIV.

In this book you will find case studies, literature reviews, experiences and lessons learned from interventions in the areas of HIV, AIDS, gender, and sexuality and education across diverse cultural contexts in the global South. We hope that these experiences will enrich your practices as you implement your projects or programmes.

Mrs Elizabeth Mataka
UN Special Envoy on HIV and AIDS in Africa

List of acronyms

ABC	Abstain, Be faithful and use Condom
AIDS	Acquired immune deficiency syndrome
AMREF	African Medical and Research Foundation
ART	Antiretroviral therapy
ASO	AIDS service organisation
BRAC	Bangladesh Rehabilitation Assistance Committee
CBO	Community-based organisation
CBVs	Community-based volunteers
CCLC	Cross-cultural Learning Conference
CSO	Civil society organisation
CWGH	Community Working Group on Health
FAWE	Forum for African Women Educationalists
FAWEU	Forum for African Women Educationalists Uganda
FBO	Faith-based organisation
FGM	Female genital mutilation
FOPHAK	Foundation of People living with HIV/AIDS in Kenya
GBV	Gender-based violence
GECPD	Galkayo Education Centre for Peace and Development
GPI	Girl Power Initiative
HBC	Home-based care
HIV	Human immunodeficiency virus
HIVOS	Humanist Institute for Development Cooperation
ICT	Information communication technology
ICW	International Community of Women Living with HIV and AIDS
IDS	Institute of Development Studies
INERELA	International Network of Religious Leaders Living with or Personally Affected by HIV or AIDS
INGO	International non-governmental organisation
ITU	International Telecommunications Union
LGBTI	Lesbian, Gay, Bisexual, Transgender and Intersex
KIT	Royal Tropical Institute
MCP	Multiple and concurrent partnership
MDG	Millennium Development Goal
M&E	Monitoring and evaluation
Mhealth	Use of mobile communication and multimedia technology for public health and well-being
MMC	Medical male circumcission
MMS	Multimedia messaging service
MSC	Most significant change
NEPAD	New Partnership for Africa's Development
NGO	Non-governmental organisation
ON	Oxfam Novib
PC	Personal computer
PDF	Portable document format
PLHIV	People living with HIV
POWA	People Opposing Women Abuse
PSI	Population Services International
RC	Resource centre
SAfAIDS	Southern Africa HIV/AIDS Information Dissemination Service
SAVE	Safe, available medication, voluntary HIV testing and empowerment through education
SMS	Short message service
SRH	Sexual and reproductive health
SRHR	Sexual reproductive health rights
SWOT	Strengths, weaknesses, opportunities and threats
ToR	Terms of reference
UAE	United Arab Emirates
UNESCO	United Nations Educational, Scientific and Cultural Organisation
UNAIDS	The Joint United Nations Programme on HIV/AIDS
UPE	Universal primary education
WHO	World Health Organisation
ZAN	Zimbabwe AIDS Network
ZITF	Zimbabwe International Trade Fair
ZNNP+	People living with HIV and AIDS in Zimbabwe

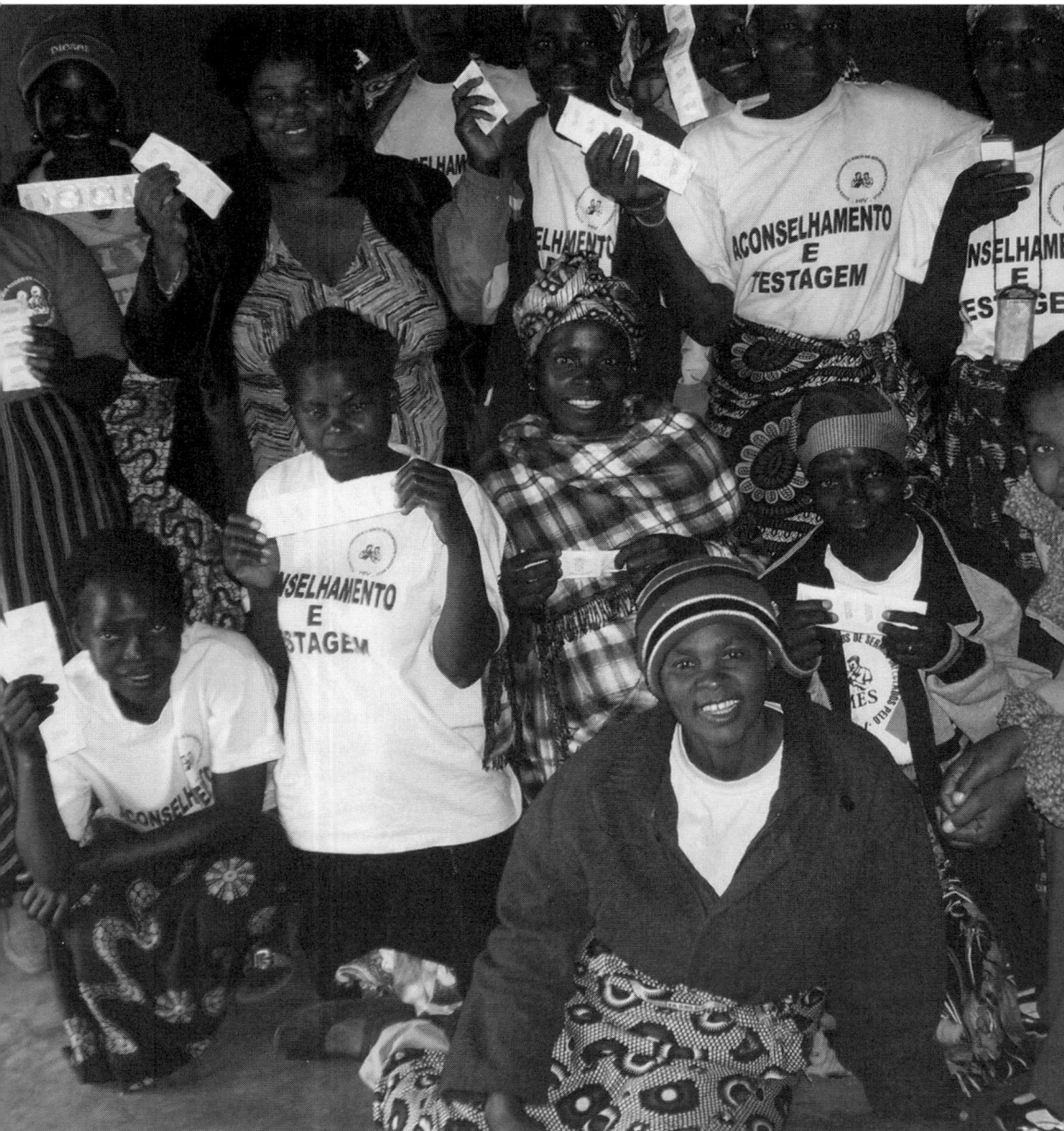

HIV and culture confluence - 'Changing the River's Flow': Possibilities and challenges in programming

Lois Chingandu, Ngoni Chibukire and Maserame Mojapele

Background information

Globalisation has shrunk the world into a virtual single community in which the actions of individuals can have global repercussions. The ever-improving accessibility to fast communications through both improved transportation and knowledge and information exchange is making this virtual community even smaller. The current global burden of diseases such as HIV, which is made worse by high incidences of gender-based violence (GBV), abuse of women's rights and harmful cultural practices, is a major concern for all. Although the global south bears the brunt of this burden and is disproportionately adversely affected, the ill-effects are felt globally. This has prompted health and development experts from both the north and south to work in partnerships to mitigate the effects of this epidemic for the mutual benefit of all.

It is against this background that SAfAIDS, in partnership with the Oxfam Novib, Hivos and KIT successfully hosted an international conference titled the 'HIV/Culture Confluence – 'Changing the River's Flow': Possibilities and Challenges in Programming on 12th and 13th April 2010'. This event was part of a four-day Cross-cultural Learning Conference.

The Cross-cultural Learning Conference was held in Johannesburg, South Africa and brought together over 130 people from Africa, Asia, Europe, the Middle East and Latin America. Delegates included health and development experts; researchers; programmers; academics and key stakeholders working in the areas of gender-based violence and HIV and AIDS; policy makers; custodians of culture and traditional leaders; and regional and international funding and technical partners (SAfAIDS, Oxfam Novib, Hivos et al., 2010).

This chapter critically analyses the topical issues presented and discussed at this conference. It also highlights key recommendations arising from deliberations. In planning this conference, SAfAIDS was of the view that in spite of the work of different stakeholders over a number of years aimed at achieving gender equality in Africa, many programme implementers and policy makers still lacked in-depth understanding and appreciation of traditional and cultural practices and their link to HIV, GBV and gender inequality in Africa.

The keynote speech at the conference focused on Africa and its growing epidemic. The presenter, Mr Sandi Mbatsha, South Africa's special advisor of Ministry of Women, Youth, Children and Persons with Disabilities, stressed that Southern Africa is the epicentre of the epidemic compared to other regions hence the need to address the fundamental underlying factors driving the epidemic. Another key speaker at the conference was Professor Michael Kelly, a Jesuit Priest, award-winning Journalist and activist. He stated:

"The conference is one that might have been less urgently needed if from the outset the response to HIV and AIDS had paid greater attention to cultural issues. But even so, after more than 28 years of trying to come to terms with the epidemic, there are now some successes: fewer people becoming infected with HIV; fewer people dying from AIDS-related causes; more than 4 million people on life-preserving antiretroviral therapy. These are significant accomplishments that we must celebrate. But as we do so, let us also remember that AIDS has not gone away. The crisis remains."

The conference was an important platform for north–south experience-sharing and information exchange as well as for fostering a deeper appreciation of multiculturalism as a reality and an important consideration in the design and implementation of HIV programmes.

Delegates were provided with opportunities to learn, not only about the socio-historical context within which HIV thrives in southern Africa, but also about the influences of culture and GBV. Delegates also discussed effective strategies to address GBV, HIV and harmful practices in cultural contexts in order to address the interlinked challenges, and lower HIV incidence in Africa and beyond.

Critical analysis of the topical issues

HIV and culture confluence: What is the evidence?
Robust discussions took place as delegates shared their views about the HIV/culture confluence. Moving from evidence to experience-based discussions, key discussants and participants had vibrant discussions on the methodologies for reducing HIV in Africa. Evidence-based confluence of HIV and cultural practices emerged as discussions moved from talking to evidence presented by Professor Michael Kelly.

Professor Michael Kelly said: "Culture is an all-pervasive concept in dealing with HIV epidemic and it is this total complex that must come into play in every meaningful response to HIV and AIDS".

The discussions led by Professor Kelly centred on the HIV/culture confluence, with focus on reflecting on the evidence that exists. The professor led delegates in an examination of the evidence of the linkages between HIV, culture and GBV. He emphasised that the issues are linked, but cautioned that programming around these issues should be linked to UNAIDS 2007 recommendations that HIV responses should be both evidence-informed and rights-based.

Participants were encouraged to shift their mindsets away from treating HIV and culture as separate entities and to realise that there is notional assent to the importance of cultural factors as key elements for understanding the local epidemic in African countries and communities. Thus the achievement of effective responses to HIV in Africa entails engaging with local lived realities of those most vulnerable to the epidemic.

Influence of cultural, social values and beliefs on HIV prevention in Africa
African countries and communities have a deep respect for culture and traditional practices, some of which have survived through generations. Mrs Elizabeth Mataka, United Nations

Special Envoy on HIV/AIDS in Africa highlighted the importance of cultural beliefs and practices in HIV prevention, given the high esteem in which many communities hold their cultures. She argued for an understanding of locally-held and valued cultural beliefs in order to positively impact on behaviour change for HIV prevention and mitigation.

"Culture is a creation of human beings who have attached a lot of meaning to it. Humans are suspended in webs of significance they themselves have spun. A failure of modernity has been the inability to grasp how people weave meaning from those webs to determine their behaviours," said Mrs Mataka.

In some cases, cultural beliefs and the practices that accompany them may actually be harmful within the context of HIV. Women and girls, who are disproportionately affected by HIV and GBV, are further marginalised by cultural arrangements that view and encourage the treatment of women as second-class citizens within their communities and homes. It is precisely because cultures present challenges to women's ability to enjoy their rights, and to protect themselves from GBV and HIV that programmers must explore culture in order to create opportunities for change and to influence attitudes and behaviour by engaging and empowering people. "Culture should not be seen as a barrier to change but as an opportunity to enhance change," Mrs Mataka asserted.

Information and communication are powerful tools in the fight against the HIV epidemic, particularly in encouraging behaviour change and engaging communities in strategising around developing culturally-sensitive HIV prevention messages. Programmers need to engage communities in message development in order to ensure that the most context-specific, culturally-sensitive information is developed and targeted effectively in order to be of the most relevance for communities. Sustainable responses can only be realised if solutions come from within.

African communities need to be encouraged to be bold enough to confront the issues driving HIV infections – if culture is killing people, it is time to confront those aspects of it and change them. Culture is dynamic. It is thus possible to challenge and shift negative aspects of cultures that increase people's vulnerability to HIV and which put others at risk. It is also entirely possible to build on positive aspects that help to prevent new infections and encourage the care and support for people living with HIV.

There is a need for a revival of the African culture of care and support to effectively deal with the stigma that surrounds HIV. Prevention must put women and girls at the centre stage to sustainably empower them to create an environment where they can protect themselves. Men should be viewed as partners: iconic men who can love without violence. African communities need to be supported to 'close the tap on new infections' by getting to the root of the spread of the epidemic, rather than continue to mop the floor without fixing the tap.

Linking HIV and culture: A missed opportunity
"People should not waste time defining culture because culture is you and me. We are a people together. Any people have a history and a context. I am because we are, since we are therefore I am" declared Professor Claude Mararike of the University of Zimbabwe.

Professor Mararike thrilled the participants with a discussion on the sociological perspective on linking HIV and culture. With reference to the research done, the main thrust of his discussion was that diseases and almost all forms of ill health are contracted and experienced within a cultural context. Thus any persons who want to advise on health issues must begin by understanding the cultural circumstances within which diseases are caused or perceived to be caused. 'Family board meetings' are traditional platforms that are effectively utilised by African people in order to discuss family matters, including disease management and mitigation.

Countries in southern Africa share a number of social and historical characteristics. For example, the majority of them experienced colonialism, which fundamentally altered and even destroyed a lot of critical aspects of their worldviews and values. "The labour migration system created during the apartheid era, for instance, has been a profound force of instability and change in African family life… The apartheid era policies not only required most couples to live apart but when one or both partners took up paid employment, actively sought to prevent them from staying together or visiting each other elsewhere," Professor Mararike added. His presentation highlighted the importance of involving family and community structures in confronting, and ultimately addressing health-related challenges, including HIV. These structures are often missed in programme implementation where organisations set up new structures instead of working with the structures and channels that are existing and comfortable for communities to use.

From Theory to practice: Key emerging issues and programme recommendations

Understanding culture

The conference also discussed religious culture, whose core is defined in three aspects related to food, sexual purity and how people relate to each other. Like traditional culture, religious culture should be understood within the local contexts in which it is experienced and practised.

"Our own culture of religion should not be static, but should change together with globalisation," stated Pastor J.P. Mokgethi-Heath of International Network of Religious Leaders Living with or Personally Affected by HIV or AIDS (INERELA). The stigma and discrimination attached to HIV emanate from fear, moral judgment, and misinformation about HIV, harmful cultures and practices, religious and moral beliefs, upbringing, superstitions and ignorance. Pastor Mokgethi-Heath maintained that there is a relationship between stigma and culture and that is why it is so difficult to deal with it. Stigma is complex; it results in a range of excluding behaviours targeted at PLHIV. It isolates, divides and breaks down family relationships and communities.

Individuals and communities need to enjoy their cultures, without worrying about contracting HIV. People also need to remember that they cannot use culture as an excuse for denying others their rights. In the context of HIV, where the fear of the epidemic lies heavily on people, many may have forgotten how to have fun, or may think that they must leave behind their cultures in order to remain HIV free. It is hoped that, among other things, people will find ideas that will help them, and the communities they serve, to celebrate their cultures safely, without infringing on the rights of others! (KIT, 2010)

Though culture is difficult to define, some researchers pointed out the misconceptions that often surround most discussion about the impact of African cultures on HIV incidence: the incorrect assumption that all African cultural practices are harmful, and the apprehensions that discussions focus almost exclusively on traditional, and mostly rural ways of living and interacting. Even though these perspectives may have their rightful place, they portray culture in a very limited and inadequate way. They fail to grasp the broad sweep of culture as comprising the myriad aspects of life that create a collective consciousness of 'how to live together'. They also fail to interrogate the positive and protective cultural practices that contribute to HIV prevention and mitigation.

The totality of what goes to make up cultural consciousness is not static but dynamic, constantly adapting to the changing external social, economic and religious environment, but at the same time modifying aspects of this environment through its interaction with them. It is this total complex that must come into play in every meaningful response to HIV and AIDS.

Culture is not a creature 'out there', culture is what people do, think, and have together. One of the cultural practices that can assist in addressing HIV is 'family board meetings'. When one member of the family is sick, the whole family is sick. When dealing with HIV, prevention and mitigation strategies should be people-driven. If the issue is not driven by the people who feel the pain, the fight is futile.

Epidemiologists attribute the different levels of HIV in urban and rural areas to the different circumstances of life in the two areas, in other words, to what are basically cultural differences between the two areas. There is enough evidence to suggest that where ways of working, playing and living together are in a 'melting pot', as is the case in many urban centres, the risk of HIV infection is higher than where there is more stability in the overall modes of life, as in most rural areas. It was recommended at the conference that more studies be conducted to clarify whether indeed this is the case.

Proposing a move to the SAVE Model of HIV prevention
INERELA's J. P. Mokhethi-Heath proposed a shift from the ABC (Abstinence, Be faithful and Condom use) approach to HIV prevention to the use of the SAVE Model. The SAVE Model is an approach to HIV prevention which was originally formulated by members of INERELA, in reaction to the shortcomings of the existing models. This approach provoked the discussions and debate on HIV prevention. Participants felt that SAVE, as a model of prevention, is biased since it only focuses on people living with HIV.

Proponents of the SAVE approach argue that it provides a more holistic way of HIV prevention by incorporating the principles of the ABC and providing additional information about HIV transmission and prevention, providing support and care for those already infected and actively challenging the denial, stigma and discrimination so commonly associated with HIV.

Used for long as the foundation of comprehensive HIV prevention programmes around the world, the ABC approach has often been presented as: 'Abstain. If you can't abstain, Be faithful. And if you can't be faithful, use a Condom'. There are arguments that the implication here is that the use of condoms automatically marks a person as being unable to be faithful, fuels stigma and acts as a disincentive to evidence-based prevention.

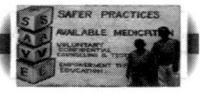

SAVE Prevention Model

S – Refers to safer practices covering all the different modes of HIV transmission, like safe blood transfusions, and the use of condoms, or sterile needles for injecting. Abstinence remains the most reliable method of avoiding exposure to STIs, but it must not be taught in isolation.

A – Refers to available medications – not just ART, but treatment for HIV-associated infections, and provision of good nutrition (particularly to help ensure adherence to ART) and clean water.

V – Refers to voluntary HIV testing and counselling. If you know you are positive, you can protect yourself and others, and take steps to live a healthy, productive, positive life.

E – Refers to empowerment through education. Denial, stigma and discrimination associated with HIV remain pernicious and ubiquitous. This is why empowerment through education is a vital component of all work on HIV. People need accurate information about HIV to make informed decisions and protect themselves, their partners and children from HIV. Education also challenges the stigma and discrimination that can make the lives of people with HIV so difficult.

Furthermore, ABC fails to consider a person's HIV status. While abstinence may be appropriate at some stages of life, at others – within a faithful marriage, for instance – it is not; and yet an HIV-negative person whose spouse is positive is at risk even within a faithful marriage. The presenter thus argued that the ABC approach is:
- Narrow – limiting itself to one mode of HIV transmission.
- Inaccurate – in assuming that people who are abstinent or faithful will completely avoid HIV, and by implying that those who are faithful do not need to use condoms as an added protective measure.
- Stigmatising to PLHIV – by implying that people who are HIV positive have failed in abstinence and faithfulness.
- Inadequate – by leaving out messages for families, communities and nations, and placing the burden of prevention on the individual.
- It ignores the role of HIV counselling, testing and treatment in prevention, and fails to highlight other measures for HIV prevention, like safe blood transfusion, safe injections, safe circumcision, and prevention of mother-to-child transmission.

How do we work together in HIV prevention in a multicultural society?
As part of the conference, SAfAIDS organised an evening culture dialogue where key discussants from the South Africa National House of Traditional Leaders, University of Zimbabwe, Sonke Gender Justice, and People Opposing Women Abuse (POWA) shared experiences on topics addressing the question "how can people work together on HIV prevention in a multicultural society?" The culture dialogues model is used by SAfAIDS as a tool for getting and providing people with information. This model was applied at the conference.

HIV and culture: "Are we talking about mixing oil and water?"
HIV and culture are not like mixing oil and water. In order to address HIV, there is a need to deal with a person holistically, and a person's culture is an integral part of who they are. Dealing with a person holistically includes not only addressing HIV as a disease that affects the person; but other diseases, such as depression, high blood pressure and diabetes. There is also a need to examine in detail whether programmers and service providers are addressing the whole person or individual parts of their body. This approach needs to be considered when addressing any disease by foregrounding the needs of the individual in their entirety, and not just their condition which needs to be overcome. This approach forgets about all those factors that go with individuals.

There is a need to address the whole person in his or her idiom, it does not help to speak to people in an idiom they do not like or identify with as the message might not come across loud and clear. "Culture is not someone or a creature out there, it is said to be people, You and Me. It is what people do, how they think and live together," Prof Mararike stated. There is no animal called culture. Family board meetings work in a way that when one family member is sick, the whole family will be sick. It is the family board that will identify the therapy required for this member. Though HIV is highly stigmatised, family board meetings can assist because a sick person might open up to one family member in particular.

Media, culture and their influence on HIV prevention
Politicians and media need to be engaged in HIV, culture and gender programming so that they do not consider HIV as merely a means of getting votes and putting themselves on the map. Media should be used as a partner in educating the community. All activists should make HIV their issue; they should not leave it to one sector of the community.

It is important to have discussions about HIV prevention and mitigation within the cultural contexts in which the people affected are located. African men, it was maintained, hide behind culture and justify negative behaviour and attitudes, some of which pose an HIV risk, by maintaining that it is 'their culture'. The fact that there is often no common understanding about culture means that people use it to benefit themselves.

Patriarchy was identified as a contributor to negative beliefs and practices. This challenge needs to be addressed. The media in its coverage of HIV should ensure that the issue of patriarchy is addressed. The media should not perpetuate the spread of the disease. There is an urgent need to educate media on how to communicate with people. The media never said anything on the issue of why men should test. There is a culture of monopoly within the media; there is a lot of control in the media whereby things are not exposed. Until this is addressed, the media will not get it right. Yet there is a need to get the media to become partners in responding to HIV and AIDS.

Merging old and new: traditional male circumcision versus medical male circumcision
There was a robust debate on issues of management of HIV and antiretroviral therapy (ART), which is an effective way of treating HIV. Given traditional beliefs and the belief in traditional healers and their remedies, discussions centred around the role of traditional healers in educating people about the use of traditional herbs when they are HIV positive. Traditional medicines, many of which work to enhance the immune system, have an important part to play in HIV treatment and management. The challenge, however, lies in the fact that a lot of these medicines are not documented and that people are not educated on their administration. Traditional healers are reluctant to share the information for fear that their intellectual property rights might be violated. Activists can assist traditional healers in preserving traditional herbs, so that important information is written down and does not get lost with the holders of the information.

Although traditional remedies have a part to play in HIV management, traditional healers need to work hand in hand with modern medical institutions so that they are able to treat the patients responsibly, and ultimately refer them to health facilities once ART initiation becomes necessary.

Medical male circumcision (MMC) demonstrates clear evidence that it is effective in reducing HIV incidence, if used in conjunction with consistent and correct condom use. There were feelings, however, that there is a need to make sure that we do not overlook the core of what circumcision is in African value systems. In the traditional context, circumcision is the cutting of the foreskin; it is initiation, a process where young men are taught how to be responsible men in their families and communities. There is a need to understand the roles of both circumcision and initiation, but also to distinguish the two and their functions in African communities. Khosi F.P. Kutama, Chairperson of the South African House of Traditional leaders, puts it succinctly: "Culture is not a problem, it is the way people interpret it. There are certain aspects in culture that need to be changed."

Traditional leaders' role in combating GBV and HIV
Culture should be approached with respect, and should be foregrounded by the identification of cultural factors that are positive and those that are negative within the context of HIV. The challenge that African societies are facing is partly due to the breakdown of cultures, and the values and social cohesion. Traditional leaders and the community at large need to be capacitated; this can be done easily and at a low cost, so that good cultural beliefs and practices are encouraged and maintained and that negative ones are challenged, and communities supported to change them. This can be done through dialogues. There is a need to motivate the traditional leaders to get involved in the fight against the epidemic.

Culture is beautiful and valuable, that is why people hold on to it; but if it is killing people, certain aspects of that culture need to be reassessed. Culture is still valuable and important, but the limitations of culture is the issue that needs to tackled.

Patriarchy and HIV infection
Patriarchy was a key issue during the discussion on the impact of culture and GBV on the prevention and spread of HIV infections. Culture and tradition are critical to sustaining the patriarchal system that has continued to subjugate and disadvantage women. Culture should be interrogated and questioned with a view to transforming societies into gender equal ones. Some believe that it is gender inequality that puts women at risk of HIV infection, and at risk of experiencing violence from their husbands, boyfriends or partners.

Patriarchal attitudes should be discouraged and gender equality and women's empowerment encouraged. As a point of departure, patriarchy should be examined so as to be able to know where power lies and what impact it has on women's bodily integrity. People should examine the power dynamics established through patriarchy with the intention of improving the system. Practices that support gender equality and gender equity should be encouraged and men should also be encouraged to challenge power imbalances perpetuated through patriarchal systems.

Patriarchy dominates people's daily cultural practices. Men are grappling with women's changing roles in the community and in the family and are resistant to change. Traditionally, altruism and ubuntu (the culture of care and support) brought about a sense of community care; individualism has replaced this. Men choose to adopt 'tough', misogynistic masculinities because of the de-masculinising process that was caused by colonialism. It seems possible that societies with strong taboos against homosexuality may motivate men to distance themselves from potential labels of gay by increasing their sexual predation and violence towards women. There is a significant link between homophobia and misogyny, since the behaviour that proves one's manhood serves both kinds of bigotry. One cannot advocate women's rights and ignore gay rights. Linking political freedom with manhood is a theme that runs strongly through the African nationalist movements.

There is a need for honest activism. For there to be positive change there is a need to do things differently by not ignoring the message those men need for self-determination and also to develop their self-esteem. There is a certain truth to the men's fear of losing their culture. Programmers should work with men to free them from the chains of their need to prove their manhood. It is no longer appropriate to claim moral neutrality; rather it is time to state clearly what kinds of approaches to HIV are acceptable to stakeholders.

Key recommendations for HIV, culture, education and gender programming from the conference

The conference came up with thirteen key recommendations for programming that emerged from the presentations, panel discussions and deliberations. The recommendations were discussed, and after a consultative process, endorsed by participants.

1. Adopt a broad definition of culture
   The conference acknowledged that culture is a difficult concept to define - however the broad definition of culture as "You and Me, the way we live, work and play together" was put forward. Culture should be defined by communities themselves, and the definitions adopted by programmers should be context and community-specific and recognise diversity.

2. Consider meaning of language
   It is important to be sensitive to the meaning and ideologies conveyed through language, thus programme implementers need to consider the use of vernacular language when developing materials and implementing programmes.

3. Role of civil society, governments and media in HIV communication
   Civil society (CS) and policy makers need to recognise the important role played by the media in socio-cultural discourse related to HIV and gender and to involve media in the processes of developing these messages. Media need to be sensitive to the messages they communicate, ensuring accuracy of terminology used (for instance use of HIV and AIDS as opposed to HIV/AIDS). Civil society should invest in ensuring that media are well capacitated to report issues accurately.

4. Consider 'our' activism
   Activism for women's rights should be integrally linked with activism for human rights, gay rights and sexual and reproductive rights. Programmers should challenge negative attitudes towards diverse sexualities (LGBTI), consider own attitudes towards LGBTI people and adopt rights-based activism and programming.

5. Aim to 'SAVE'
   Consider, in the response, multiple and concurrent partnerships (MCP), male circum-

cision (MC), drugs and alcohol and intergenerational sex as key drivers of HIV. Promote SAVE as a strategy for HIV prevention as it is more holistic and responsive to the socio-cultural context in which we live, if we are to 'close the tap' on new infections.

6. Respect and involve traditional leadership
Greater impact can be achieved when traditional leaders are sensitised, engaged and involved in high-level policy meetings at regional level. Traditional leaders can be proactive in approaching civil society, if they have work-plans; it is easier for CS to identify where the intervention is needed and areas of collaboration.

7. Respect the value of culture in HIV and gender programmes
Ensure respect for the capacity of communities themselves to address negative cultural practices and encourage positive/protective cultural practices.

8. Recognise the multi-factoral nature of HIV transmission
Consider that HIV is not just about sex, but also may be influenced by genetics, social environment, political context, economics as well as culture. Greater effort is needed to gather evidence and understand the local epidemic. 'Know Your Epidemic' - studies should push the boundaries to understand all factors driving HIV.

9. Discourage patriarchal attitudes and encourage gender equality and women's empowerment
Understand patriarchy and the contexts in which it occurs. The power dynamics established through patriarchy need to be examined with the intention of improving the system. Male participation in challenging power imbalances perpetuated through patriarchal systems should be encouraged.

10. Develop indicators which monitor changes in gender and cultural practices which influence HIV
While it is difficult to measure complex factors, programmes need to identify mechanisms to monitor changes in practice that influence HIV. Consider qualitative approaches to the collection of information and to supporting documentation within communities. There is a need to document existing good cultural practices to support our work within cultural contexts.

11. Civil society should be firm and principled while addressing culture
Civil society should communicate/do advocacy work focusing on policy makers, donors and relevant stakeholders to communicate the value of a cultural approach to HIV and gender programmes.

12. Engaging young people and the impact of education in HIV mitigation
Voices of young people need to be heard more at regional and international platforms. Focus should be on encouraging inter-generational dialogue. Education must be offered by various stakeholders and through various approaches such as schools, medical services, family, media and peers to reinforce the message of gender, education and HIV.

13 Religion, HIV and gender work
   Understand the role that religious culture plays in contemporary societies.

Conclusion

As AIDS service organisations, we need to make efforts to build the capacity of communities by helping them to understand how culture is linked to gender inequality, HIV, GBV, education, among others. Let us encourage them to focus only on how to address the negative aspects of their diverse cultures while promoting positive ones. As Professor Michael Kelly aptly put it: "Culture is an all-pervasive concept in dealing with HIV epidemic and it is this total complex that must come into play in every meaningful response to HIV and AIDS". Let us remember this as we make interventions in diverse cultural contexts.

References

KIT. *Exchange on HIV and AIDS, Sexuality and Gender* magazine, June, 2010.
SAfAIDS, Oxfam Novib, Hivos and KIT. "HIV/Culture Confluence." Conference, Johannesburg, South Africa, 2010, April 12 to 15.

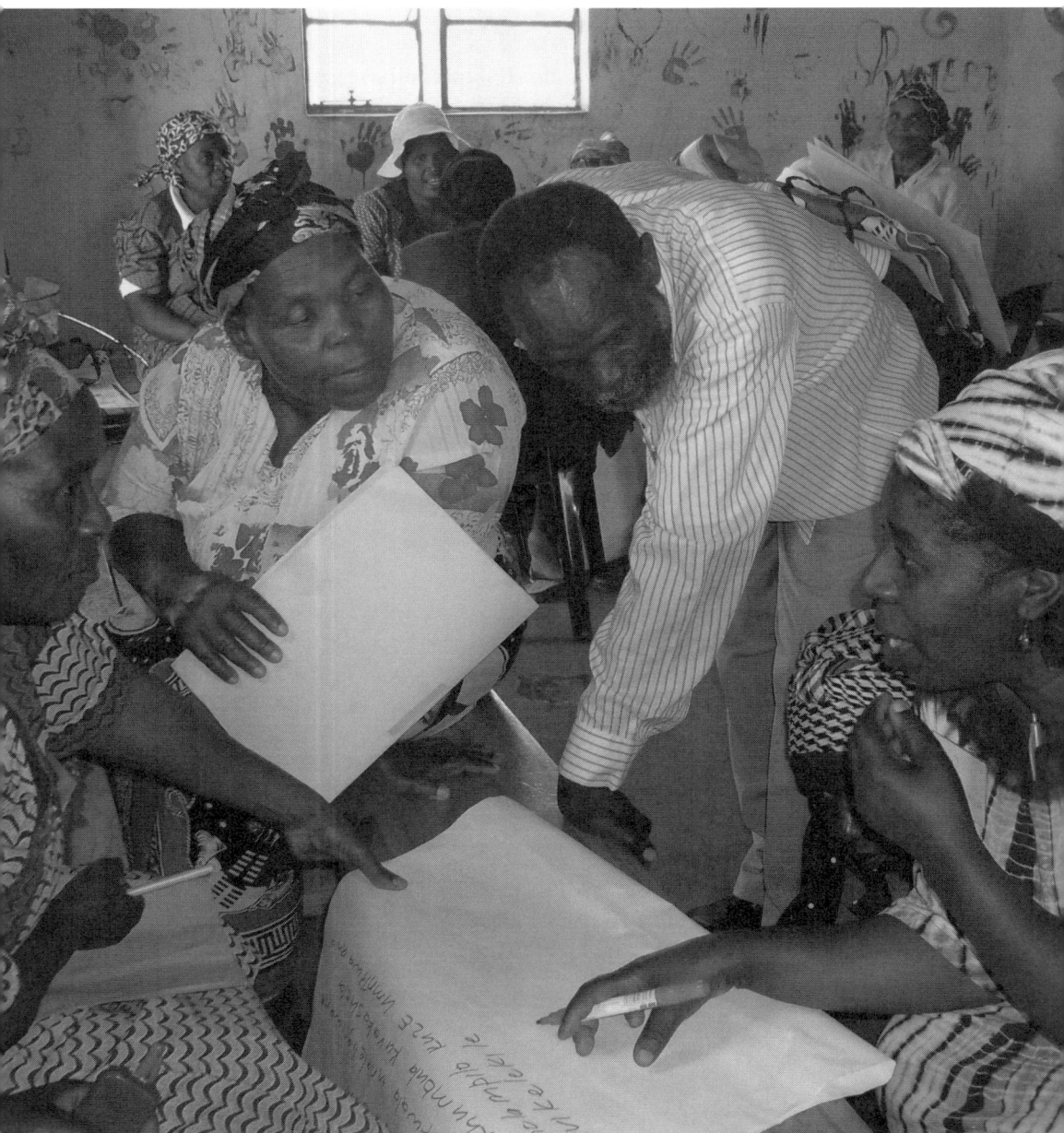

SAfAIDS Changing the River's Flow Model: A social ecological behaviour change intervention for HIV prevention in southern Africa

Lois Chingandu, Ngoni Chibukire and Maserame Mojapele

Southern Africa is now in the third decade of the HIV epidemic. According to the UNAIDS 2008 report about 33.4 million people are living with HIV, of which 70% are from Sub-Saharan Africa. About 60% of those infected are women. The rates of gender-based violence (GBV) are quite alarming; one in every five women has been abused in one way or another. This shows that HIV and GBV incidences have a woman's face in Africa. Women are the worst affected and infected, yet they carry the overall burden of caring for the sick, orphans and vulnerable children.

The response to the epidemic has therefore been multi-sectoral, with governments, non-governmental organisations (NGOs) and community-based organisations (CBOs) working together in mounting a response. At both regional and national levels, various policy instruments, codes, strategic frameworks, plans and legal documents are in place that stakeholders are using in rolling out their interventions. There have been some successes achieved, with countries like Kenya, Uganda, Zambia and Zimbabwe recording reductions in HIV prevalence rates during the past few years. However, rates, and in particular incidence rates, still remain unacceptably high in southern Africa, hence the need to scale-up the implementation of programmes that are owned by communities and implemented by community members themselves. These interventions need to be locally-driven and culturally-sensitive for positive behaviours to be realised and maintained.

The patriarchal arrangement of the majority of communities in southern Africa has been identified as a major contributing factor to women's subordinate position, lack of agency and consequently to their susceptibility to GBV and HIV; this continues to undermine efforts to attain Millennium Development Goal Three (MDG 3 which seeks to promote gender equality and empower women), and to effectively respond to the epidemic. Although various countries have enacted laws criminalising GBV, and set out penalties for offenders, the fact that most incidences of GBV occur in the private sphere in the form of domestic violence means that it is difficult to police, and that violence against women and girls will persist within communities in the region. There have been links made between women's vulnerability to violence and their increased susceptibility to contracting HIV, and women's increased chances of experiencing various forms of violence if they are HIV positive.

Women and girls are the worst affected by both GBV and HIV, the human rights of women and girls are the most violated, and socio-economically, culturally and politically, women are the most disempowered due to the gender inequalities that persist in African societies. The key question is then, how are all these violations of women interrelated?
The key outcomes of gender inequality, violation and limited access to rights for women

are increased GBV and greater susceptibility to contracting HIV transmission. It is important to note that:
- Gender-based violence, whether it is physical, financial, mental or emotional, and culturally-supported inequalities between men and women, leading to unequal sexual relationships, contribute to risky sexual behaviours that place women and girls at greater risk of HIV infection.
- Women who disclose their HIV positive status may be subjected to brutal beatings, abuse, assault, abandonment and accused of being promiscuous and shameless.
- Misconceptions and beliefs can also result in the spread of HIV, particularly the belief that having sex with a virgin girl can cure AIDS. This perception puts girls and young women at risk of being raped by people living with HIV, hence increasing HIV incidence, and unwanted pregnancies among this demographic.
- Both GBV and HIV involve the violation of the rights of women and girls. Women's rights are human rights and should be upheld at all times. Women's enjoyment of their rights to dignity and sexual and reproductive health are limited in southern Africa.

Why have we failed to reduce women's vulnerability to HIV and GBV in Africa?
While it is universally agreed that cultural practices and structures play a central role in driving the epidemic, this has not necessarily translated into any meaningful intervention at policy and programming levels. Instead many interventions that have been promoted for years, like the ABC approach, have not reduced women's vulnerability to HIV and GBV. This approach does not, to a large extent, address the socio-cultural factors that are worsening the twin epidemics. Both policy makers and programmers continue to shy away from designing interventions that directly focus on the fundamentals of cultural beliefs and practices that are driving the epidemic. Some believe and assert that these are rigid systems that cannot change.

The work of SAfAIDS through the Changing the River's Flow (CTRF) interventions, which are hinged on many theories, have demonstrated that African cultures do change when confronted with threats to life, in this case HIV. Such change can only take place if custodians of culture are committed, involved directly and communities are empowered to become agents of change. Programmes usually fail because 'outsiders' inappropriate solutions for problems. For programmes to be effective, communities should be empowered to identify their own problems and appropriate solutions to tackle such challenges.

A cultural approach to addressing HIV in southern Africa:
A groundbreaking intervention?
Given the evidence that women who experience domestic violence are at greatest risk of being infected with HIV due to lack of agency and power to negotiate for safer sex among other factors, Lois Chingandu and Neddy Matshalaga (2004) figure 1, developed an integrated model that addresses the linkages between GBV, culture, women's rights and HIV, as depicted in the flow chart below.

In this model Chingandu and Matshalaga advocate for the adoption of a comprehensive integrated approach when addressing GBV, culture and HIV. Studies indicate that employing vertical programming around these issues is not effective. It is more effective to address the issues in a balanced and holistic manner, without blaming men or women, but by

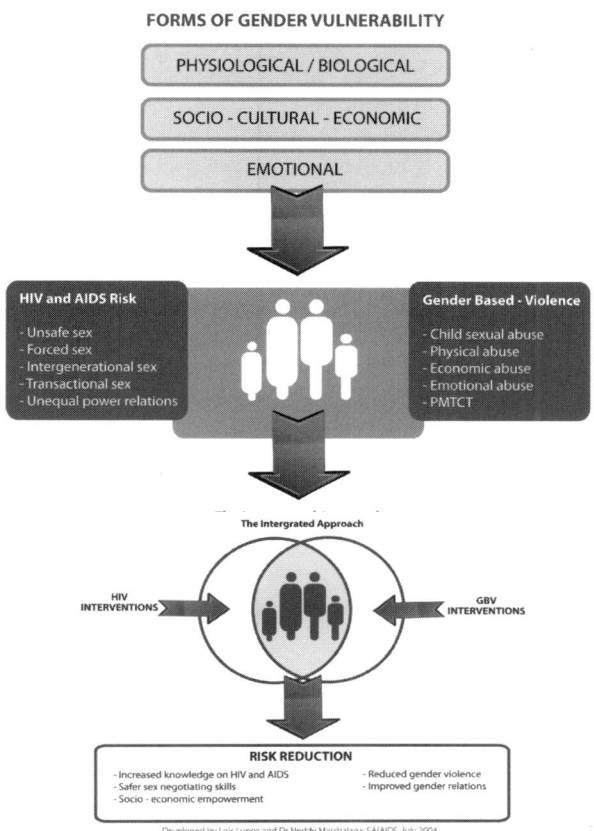

Figure 1: An integrated model that addresses the linkages between GBV, culture, women's rights and HIV

working with both sexes together in order to discuss the identified problems and to identify amicable community-oriented solutions that will translate into individual behaviour change and community social transformation.

Initiation of the 'Changing the River's Flow' Programme

A large powerful river has sprung from a small tributary originating in Seke, a peri-urban community located 50 kilometres southeast of Harare, the capital city of Zimbabwe. The river meanders swiftly across nine southern African countries, providing life-saving tools and strategies for survival to rural and urban communities alike.

The metaphor of a river helps to explain the birth, growth and reach of SAfAIDS' flagship programme, the 'Changing the River's Flow programme', a uniquely African intervention that sees programmers and stakeholders in southern Africa confronting harmful cultural practices and GBV in order to prevent HIV and to reduce incidence rates in the region.

The programme, which was piloted in Seke in 2006, before being scaled up to other countries and communities, has been recognised by a selection committee set up in Zimbabwe and was documented as a Best Practices in HIV prevention and mitigation.

This project was implemented to address some of the harmful cultural practices that are still common and that increase women's vulnerability to HIV and GBV. Certain cultural norms have been shown to dis-empower women in Africa, silencing their voices and contributing to the HIV crisis by preventing women from acting to protect themselves and their families. Acknowledging that communities in southern Africa must act in order to make their cultures safe to practice within the context of HIV is an important first step; but knowing how to deal with these problems is not always self-evident. It is therefore important to enhance communities' capacity and help them to creatively imagine, dream up and implement solutions and alternatives that are life-affirming and which they can sustain.

This is one of the reasons why the 'Changing the River's Flow' metaphor was adopted as the theme for the programme, it was hoped that this metaphor would encourage the 'dream work' that must necessarily accompany work around culture and HIV.

Figure 2: The 'Changing the River's Flow' logo, showing a person swimming against the course of the river to prevent HIV

The choice of the image of a flowing river was chosen because culture is a bit like a river. Picture a large, powerful river with rapids, some permanent waves and whirlpools. Most likely, all the people in the neighbourhood know the rapids and some may earn a living from their knowledge by helping others cross safely. According to Dr Leigh Price, who coined the metaphor:

> …the river has its moods depending on the seasons, but for the most part it is predictable. It has always been like this. Or has it? In fact, geology tells us that rivers change and their 'permanency' is often a trick of our perception, based on our short human lifespan. In the same way, culture may seem mostly permanent, but this is a trick of our perception. Culture is always changing and adjusting to different circumstances. If there is a cultural norm that is problematic from an HIV point of view, communities might want to remove it. Laws can be enacted to prevent it or it can be scooped out, but it will tend to reform unless people address the underlying causes of it, such as poverty and misogyny. There is no way a river could flow upstream but it can be diverted in one way or the other as it continues its downstream flow. Culturally things can be done differently in a positive and sustainable way.

On the other hand, it is important to view a river as a source of life and object of beauty. Culture is both a necessary part of life, beautiful and valuable in itself. Therefore, communities should be reminded to be respectful of culture and to celebrate its richness and diversity, even if, at the same time, there is consensus that certain aspects of culture are not progressive in the era of HIV and AIDS, hence the need to transform them in a locally-driven and culturally-sensitive manner.

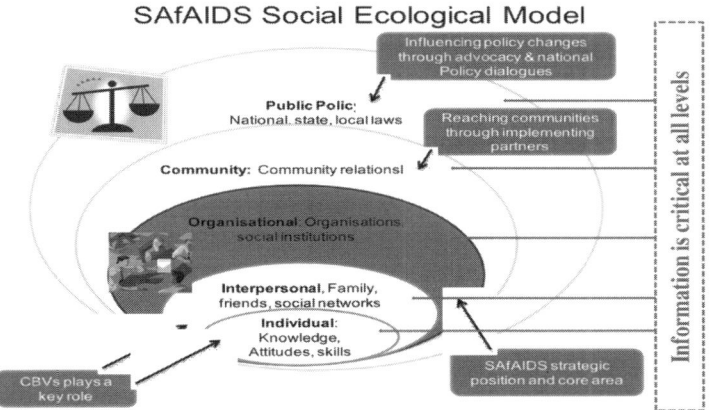

Figure 3: SAfAIDS-Adapted Social Ecological Model of Behaviour Change

From theory to practice: A Social-ecological model/approach to the Changing the River's Flow Programme

It is important to note at this stage that the 'Changing the River's Flow' programme is a behaviour change intervention that has its basis in theoretical models of individual behaviour change. The programme follows a Social Ecological Behaviour Change Model that SAfAIDS adapted as illustrated above.

The core assumption under this Model is that behaviour change is a multivariate equation that is determined by several factors, and which is experienced within a specific environment and context, and as such interventions should aim at tackling all the factors involved - from the individual to policy levels. McLeory, BiBeau, Steckler and Glanz (1988) proposed a Health Behaviour Change Model, from which the Social Ecological Model was adapted, that intervenes on five levels of influence: at the intrapersonal, interpersonal processes and primary groups, institutional factors, community factors and public policy. This Model also takes into account individual and environmental factors. What makes SAfAIDS' 'Changing the River's Flow' programme effective is that it focuses on these multiple social layers and on behaviour change as caused by various factors. The expected behaviour changes take place at individual, community and policy levels.

The results framework (see figure 4) as developed by Chingandu and Chrispin Chomba (2010) shows various anticipated changes at each level of intervention. The long-term impact would be a reduction in risky behaviours and thus reduced HIV incidence rates in southern Africa.

Description of the CTRF model; key principles of the intervention

The 'Changing the River's Flow' model is based on eight key principles that should be considered in implementing this programme. The critical considerations include:
- Appreciating that HIV is a complex matter, and that some cultural practices have now become risky and threatening to life;
- Recognising that individual change is not sustainable unless focus is placed on community change through systematic and consistent dialogue;
- Understanding that certain cultural practices play a decisive role in fuelling women's rights violations, and subsequently the HIV epidemic;

- Recognising the critical triple linkage between culture, HIV and women's rights;
- Cognisance that not all cultural practices and norms are 'bad', and that there are positive components of cultural structures that can be harnessed to reverse vulnerability of women and girls, within the context of HIV;
- Recognition that the solutions lie within the communities, who understand their culture best, and thus hold the reins of 'cultural transformation';
- The understanding that changing the direction of culture (symbolised as the 'river') is not synonymous with rejecting culture as a whole (the 'river' should be left to flow but in a different direction);
- Acknowledging that cultural norms and values are vital and should be preserved within a milieu that does not enhance HIV-related risk and vulnerability (adapted from a booklet, A Path to Sustained Change through Culture Dialoguing- Chingandu and Eghtessadi, 2009)

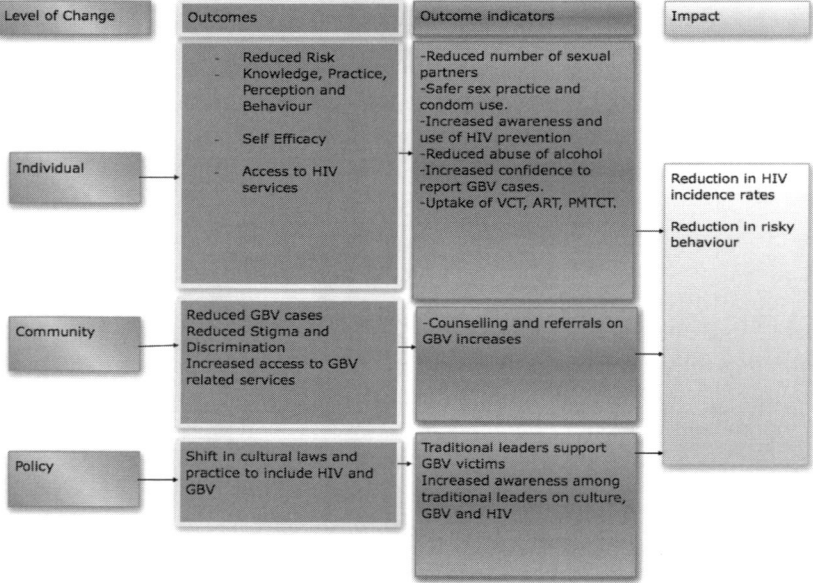

Figure 4: A results framework for the CTRF Programme

Key strategic components of the CTRF programme

The key question that programmers continue to ask is whether this approach to HIV programming can really make a difference in southern Africa. Can traditional leadership and communities transform their ways of doing things and their belief systems, thus impacting on the ways in which they practice their cultures?

If we are to adopt the definition of culture shared by Professor Claude Mararike (2010) as "you and me"; there is nothing that can stop the 'two' from addressing the cultural issues that negatively affect them and that are counter-progressive. As a collective, the 'two' can be encouraged to discuss and reach consensus on contentious issues and to agree on the way forward.

Through its innovative and creative approaches to programming under the 'Changing the River's Flow' programme, SAfAIDS developed six key pillars of intervention to ensure an effective and holistic response to the HIV epidemic in southern Africa. In the years to come the programme is expected to continue to make a substantial impact in the fight against GBV, harmful cultural practices, violation of women's rights and HIV incidence.

The six strategies include:

1. Leadership sensitisation, community mobilisation and understanding of the community-specific interactions of the linkages through baseline assessments in targeted communities.
2. Conducting culturally-acceptable and community-led dialogues, with the 'outsider organisations' playing a facilitative role.
3. Organising appropriate community-based capacity development activities to respond to the needs of community members as expressed by them during the dialogues and other interventions.
4. Conducting capacity building activities for Community-Based Volunteers, who are the change agents.
5. Supporting partners and communities with relevant and up-to-date community-oriented materials.
6. Facilitating community outreach programmes through door-to-door campaigns or face-to-face interactions by change agents at community level.

Leadership sensitisation, community mobilisation and baseline assessments

'Leadership' includes traditional leaders such as chiefs, village headmen, local councillors and political and religious leaders in a community. Different countries may use different names and titles but these are the decision-makers who oversee community projects and other day-to-day activities. Implementing the 'Changing the River's Flow' programme requires strong leadership endorsement, commitment and buy-in for the programme to be effective. The buy-in of community leaders can be achieved through conducting leadership sensitisation meetings and having informal meetings and discussions with influential people in the community prior to, and during programme roll-out. If community leaders understand the nature and focus of the programme, as well as the intended outcomes, they are more likely to be supportive.

Baseline assessments and community mobilisation can only be done if traditional leaders are agreeable to the interventions; their participation has been shown to be crucial to the inclusion and retention of community members during programme implementation. When community leaders lead from the front, by participating in community meetings and dialogues, the programme is more likely to be well received by community members, and to achieve some real, and sustainable change. It is important that the community feels a sense of ownership of the programme. They should not feel that it has been imposed upon them; efforts should be made to convince them that their common problems require solutions that work best when discussed, agreed on and endorsed by all community members. This thus entails encouraging communities to identify challenges and problems in their own communities, and to find their own solutions to these problems.

Conducting culturally-acceptable community dialogues

Community dialogues are friendly platforms that are created to discuss pertinent issues that affect communities, with the ultimate objective of finding sustainable and context-specific solutions. Participants in the dialogues are not dictated to but are rather given opportunities to discuss issues among themselves, with the intention of finding lasting solutions.

The community dialogue approach has been found to be the preferred African way of discussing community problems, building consensus and finding community-specific solutions. According to Professor Mararike of the University of Zimbabwe, such discussions are done through what has been coined traditional 'family board meetings', where family members come together to discuss and find solutions to issues and challenges, from pending marriages, ill-health and financial matters to death, among others. Since time immemorial, this approach has been working effectively and remains functional today.

In order to achieve the most impact, the community dialogues are held in 'rounds'. SAfAIDS has found that in order to be effective, it is best to hold the first 'rounds' with men only, women only and custodians of culture and traditional leaders only. Due to cultural sensitivities attached to discussing sex and sexuality, and violence, which are often considered as taboo or 'private matters' which are not to be discussed in public, the separation of the sexes allows people to be more open and vocal in identifying issues that fuel HIV in their communities. It is also useful to have mixed groups of very young girls and older women, as cultural barriers are also age-determined. It is also useful to separate the sexes because typically, in the first rounds women and men will tend to blame each other for the HIV and GBV incidences identified as problems in the community.

Community facilitators (project staff who are well known and respected, and who often live in the community) are ideally placed to provide an entry-point to getting communities to talk, and in leading the dialogues and providing relevant information on HIV and GBV. In the second 'rounds' of dialogues, the groups are brought together in order to discuss issues identified from the first 'rounds' of dialogues. Issues raised are linked to gender, GBV, women's rights and HIV. The discussions at this stage are reinforced by use of performing arts, which helps to depersonalise some harmful cultural practices happening in the community, allowing community members to identify and realise the risky practices that contribute to high HIV and GBV incidences in their communities. During these rounds, individuals realise that there is a problem, and they become more open to changing behaviour in order to ensure that they protect themselves and their families from HIV and GBV. The facilitator leading the dialogues at this point should be knowledgeable about the linkages.

The third 'rounds' are held in separate groups again. Women and men's groups both focus on HIV, gender, culture and women's rights but the focus is also on discussing how each sex is affected by these variables. Custodians of culture consider and discuss the link between cultural laws and practices and how these negatively impact on the lives of women and girls in their community within the context of HIV. The community is then better prepared for discussions about solutions to the challenges they experience in the final 'rounds' of dialogue.

The final 'rounds' of dialogue are more action-oriented. During these rounds community members hold more discussions on issues they would have identified in the previous 'rounds.' They are encouraged to identify their own capacity gaps and to find solutions that can be used to address some of these issues. The discussions may be tense as people try to find solutions, and to reach consensus on the way forward and to come up with clear, sustainable solutions to community problems. In the end it is worth it as communities identify strategies to prevent HIV while still enjoying their cultures. As highlighted above these dialogues are repeated several times. The community dialogue framework (see figure 5) shows how these dialogues progress from round one to the last round.

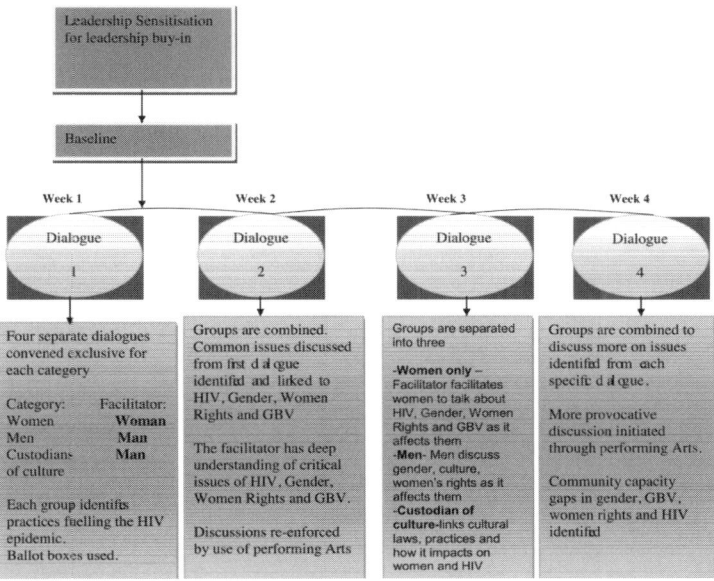

Figure 5: A community dialogue framework developed by Chomba and Chingandu (2010)

Organising appropriate community-based capacity development activities

Given the magnitude of the HIV epidemic, it is critical to improve communities' capacities to respond to the epidemic. Based on baseline findings and also on problems/challenges identified during community dialogues, communities are offered opportunities to participate in various capacity development and enhancement activities. Capacity development areas include training in risk reduction strategies, couple's communication, GBV and HIV prevention, sex and sexuality, condom use, customary law, and traditional practices and policies that have implications on gender equality and HIV transmission.

Conducting capacity building activities for Community-Based Volunteers

Communities need people who steer and drive programme activities at local level through door-to-door or face-to-face interactions. These community change agents are commonly referred to as Community-Based Volunteers (CBVs) in the 'Changing the River's Flow' programme. Community-Based Volunteers are selected from within the community and are people who can "walk the talk". In order for CBVs to effectively deliver, they are also empowered with important information on gender, culture, women's rights and HIV transmission. They are also provided with materials for dissemination and monitoring tools that they use for tracking purposes. They are offered on-going mentoring and periodically targeted for additional training in other pertinent issues as the need arises.

Supporting partners and communities with relevant and up-to-date community-oriented materials

As part of programme support, SAfAIDS provides CBVs and implementing partners with relevant and up-to-date materials for distribution at local level. The materials provided reinforce the information received during training. SAfAIDS encourages partners to translate materials and information that is relevant for their communities into local languages.

Community outreach programmes

The door-to-door campaigns approach has proven to be a cost-effective way of targeting and disseminating information; community change agents disseminate information door-to-door to the most appropriate audiences. Community-Based Volunteers also conduct focus groups discussions and can offer referrals to specialised services where needed, as they often have strong links with the local New Start Centre, clinic, domestic violence unit at the police station and with the religious and community leaders in communities in which they operate. New Start Centres are a Population Services International (PSI) initiative and that's where people are counselled and tested. Each CBV can reach out to as many as 20 people per month, which translates into about 240 people reached per year. SAfAIDS has approximately 10,000 CBVs working in various communities in Lesotho, Namibia, Mozambique, South Africa, Swaziland, Zambia and Zimbabwe.

Stories of Change: Is 'Changing the River's Flow' Making a Difference?

In concluding this chapter it is important to examine whether the programme has made an impact since it has grown into a regional programme. Anecdotal evidence shows that the programme is making a difference in countries where the programme is being implemented. Below are some of the outcomes that have been realised to date.

Greater openness and increased dialogue among community members

A programme beneficiary in Malawi noted that:

> "Prior to the cultural dialogues there was not much information about GBV, culture, HIV and women's rights. Now thanks to the dialogues communities can adequately link the issues. Sometimes it is just about people not having enough information."

This indicates that the creation of platforms for dialogue is critical for the sharing of information and for discussing issues in a non-confrontational manner, and also that information has the power to make a difference. In Malawi community members managed to reach a consensus to ban polygamy, but the only complication was that the Chief had three wives, which put him in a dilemma.

Increased acceptance of and demand for condom use among married couples

In Seke Rural Community (Zimbabwe), where the project was piloted in 2006/7, married couples were trained on risk reduction strategies, including condom use. As part of telling the stories of change, one woman explained that:

> "...the fact that we attended the same course and dialogues with my husband and were given the same information has made it easy to discuss sex and negotiate condoms".

Usually married couples do not use condoms in many African societies, so the reported acceptance and uptake of condoms by this demographic is a major breakthrough for the programme, and for HIV prevention efforts.

Enhanced communication around sex and sexuality issues

It is a taboo to talk about sex and sexuality issues in many communities. Dialogue, information material support and capacity development activities around sex and sexuality issues can open avenues for communication on issues that used to be taboo. Women are now free to discuss condom use as part of support group services.

Increased access to relevant information about HIV-related issues

One of the pillars of the CTRF programme is material production and dissemination at community level during dialogues, community events and other activities. One unmarried female youth in Seke Community was quoted as saying:

> "…before, I did not want to say yes, but I had to, because I did not have the knowledge, now I know I have the rights, I know what is safe and I can say 'no' if I want."

This is a powerful message which shows how women can be empowered through information to make their own decisions on sexual matters.

Changing harmful cultural practices

Through dialogue, communities can be encouraged to identify those cultural practices that do not promote gender equality and which create fertile ground for the transmission of HIV. After the dialogues, some communities report that there is growing disapproval of cultural practices that pose an HIV risk, such as wife inheritance, "small houses" - a common practice whereby men have additional sexual partners whom they maintain in a second household, even raising families with them, and polygamy since they put women and men at increased risk of HIV infection. In places where these practices are still common, people are doing them differently, often by getting tested for HIV before commitments are made.

Success story of the Changing the Rivers Flow

"I was married to a man who everyone knew had many other partners. When he went away to work for a time, I knew he would not be faithful. So, when he returned home I told him he must use a condom, but he refused. I went to the headman and told him my problem. The headman agreed with me and spoke to my husband, asking him to use a condom. My husband refused, and in the end I had to divorce him and the headman agreed. My husband has since died, so if I had stayed with him, I would also be dead." Woman from Seke.

Traditionally, it is taboo for a woman to divorce her husband. Neither of the families will allow it. Dialogues and community interventions have empowered women to overturn such beliefs. It is important to note that the woman had the support of the local leadership and the community itself to take such a decision. This shows how powerful this model is in transforming certain beliefs and practices in communities in southern Africa.

Conclusion

Cultural transformation requires time and commitment, even in the face of resistance, if sustained change is to be achieved. Communities' engagement in culture, HIV and gender-related issues should be an ongoing process that will enable them to find 'solutions that fit' their specific contexts and situations. Africa can reverse the course of the HIV epidemic if programmers and communities address the fundamental socio-cultural factors that are driving the epidemic. An African problem calls for African solutions.

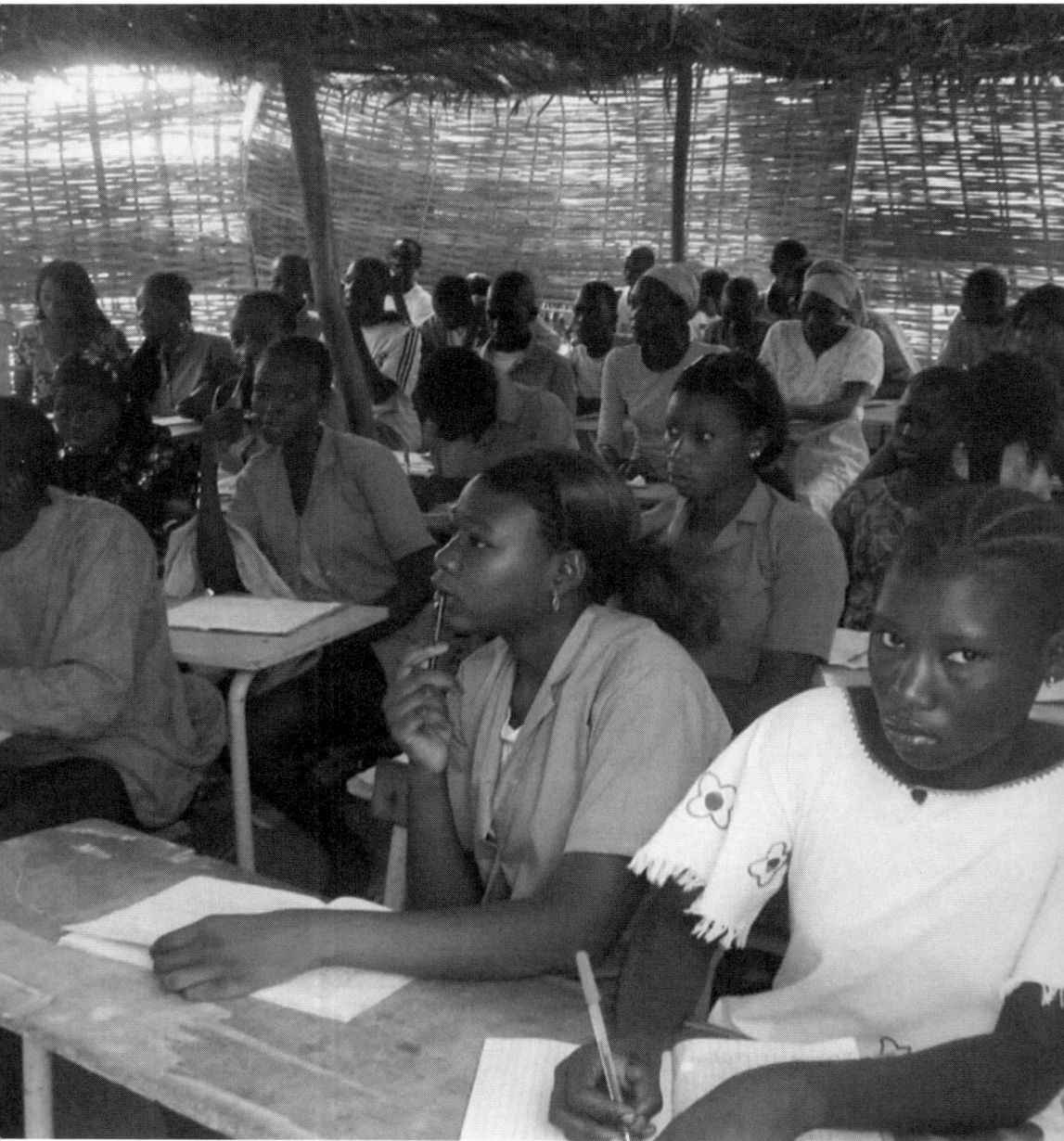

The Innovation Fund: Supporting education, gender and HIV prevention

Olloriak Sawade and Jeanette Kloosterman

Introduction
Oxfam Novib (ON) puts five basic rights at the core of all its work.[1] Those rights are mutually connected and cannot be treated separately. ON is of the opinion that a combined approach to gender justice, education and HIV and AIDS offers an aggregated value and important advantages, which in the end will lead to more gender justice, good quality education and less HIV and AIDS prevalence. It is for this reason that ON established the Innovation Fund in 2007 to promote original new projects with a combined focus on education, gender, and HIV.[2] The Innovation Fund totalled 26 million Euros and funded over 100 different projects around the world. The Fund was a pilot project and was based on temporary resources; therefore it came to an end in 2010. However, the concepts, lessons learned and innovations will continue through ON's regular programming.

This chapter is written for practitioners working around education, gender justice and HIV prevention with the hope that others can learn from the experiences of the Fund. The chapter examines the Innovation Fund theoretically and practically; the importance and relevance of the interconnection between the prevention of HIV and AIDS, education and gender justice will be analysed and lessons learned and challenges encountered will be discussed. Throughout the chapter you will find short reviews of Innovation Fund projects that illustrate the innovative character of the interventions connected to our theoretical supposition.

Oxfam Novib's application of the Innovation Fund Triangle
For ON it is clear that it is important to connect the work of women's rights organisations in raising consciousness about gender inequality with the work of educational institutions (formal and informal) and HIV and AIDS organisations.
The issues of gender equality and prevention of HIV could be promoted in educational organisations. To be effective, HIV and AIDS organisations cannot deny the problems surrounding HIV infection and AIDS, nor the fact that these are connected to gender justice issues and vice versa. For this reason, women's rights organisations could include HIV and AIDS as a topic in their programmes of action, something which is not often the case. In short, without taking a holistic view of gender justice, HIV and education, important opportunities may be lost.

---

[1] The right to 1. sustainable livelihoods, 2. essential services (health, water, education), 3. rights in crisis, 4. political participation and 5. identity (gender and diversity).

[2] Although HIV prevention is a major component to the Fund within most projects funded, HIV prevention is part of a much larger program of Sexual Reproductive Health Rights (SRHR).

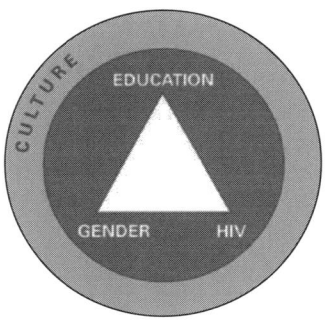

Why Gender Justice issues?
Oxfam Novib defines *gender justice* as the ending of the inequalities between men and women, which in most cases is the end of the subordination of women to men. The notion 'gender' makes it possible to distinguish the biological, sexual differences between women and men from the socio-cultural differences. The biological differences cannot be changed; they have the character of destination. But culturally-determined differences are the functions and roles adopted or received by men and women respectively in a certain society. These differences can be transformed, and vary according to political influences and the evolution of opinion (Ostergaard, 1991). Today ON, and with it many other organisations and people, wish to fight the inequality that stems from a patriarchal gender ideology which for centuries has lain at the centre of human socialisation worldwide. This means that ON believes in the possibility of changing cultural constructs and traditions and that, in order to do that, men and boys have to be involved in this change process. This helps to see gender justice as an outcome and as a process.

In the context of the Innovation Fund, gender justice, as an outcome, means equal access to good quality education, health and the self-determination of women in their sexuality, reproduction and lives or lifestyles, which implies, amongst other things, that women are free from gender-based violence (GBV)[3] and are empowered. Gender justice, as a process, brings in the essential element of accountability, which implies the responsibility and answerability of precisely those social institutions set up to dispense justice: that can be the State through laws, school, family, community and religious groups. In one way or another, these institutions are supposed to settle disputes, establish and enforce laws, and prevent the abuse of power. Understanding the ideological and cultural justifications for women's subordination within each arena can help identify how to challenge patterns of gender inequality (Goetz, 2007).

Ironically it is often exactly those institutions where cultural and patriarchal ideas about gender equality are reproduced. However, this means that they could also play a role in challenging them. In the family, for example, during primary socialisation processes it is often the mother herself who communicates the subordination and discrimination of

---

[3] ON follows the UN-definition of GBV, mentioned in the Declaration on the Elimination of Violence against Women (1993): "any act of gender-based violence that results in, or is likely to result in physical, sexual or psychological harm or suffering to women, including threats of such acts, coercion or arbitrary deprivation of liberty, whether occurring in public or private life." The Declaration refers to physical, sexual and psychological violence, wherever it occurs (art. 1+2).

women. Afterwards this process is reinforced by secondary socialisation processes that take place at school, but also in religious institutions, the community and the wider public domain (Antrobus, 2004). This takes us to the role educational institutions play in the reproduction of gender inequality patterns and stereotypical thinking. ON believes that families and schools are crucial entry points for the realisation of increased justice in gender relations, hence less violence against women and girls and the prevention of HIV and AIDS (Antrobus, 2004 and Restrepo Ramirez, 1992).

To show a practical example one can look at Somalia where gender discrimination is widespread. Somali women have little opportunity to benefit from education (including sexuality education), political and economic participation and decision-making. They are for the most part restricted to household chores and marginal positions in their communities. Existing cultural and traditional structures within the society favour boys and men at the expense of women. In order for women and girls to rise above these challenges and participate in the reconstruction of the Somali state, education and knowledge of how to protect their own bodies is of paramount importance.

The Innovation Fund supported the Galkayo Education Centre for Peace and Development (GECPD), a Somali organisation, in order to develop an education programme that focuses on gender, HIV, AIDS, GBV and female genital mutilation (FGM), which is particularly relevant to the cultural context. The programme specifically targeted primary and secondary schools, youth groups and non-formal family life education centres. Part of the training involved educating primary and secondary teachers and representatives from the community, including religious leaders and politicians on issues concerning gender and Sexual Reproductive Health Rights (SRHR). The project specifically targeted the cultural and traditional structures that exist in Somalia in order to try and reform current societal thinking that disempowers women.

There are many innovative aspects to this project. The GECPD project was able to create space to discuss a sensitive issue like FGM in public and to include religious and political leaders within the community. This project learned from a similar Innovation Fund project in Nigeria that works with Islamic religious leaders and that has learned many lessons itself, e.g. about what language to use when discussing issues around sexuality and what passages within the Koran should be highlighted when discussing with (and convincing) Islamic leaders the importance of education for girls and information about the prevention of HIV.

Good quality education helps

In its position paper on education, ON defines "good quality education" as education that leads to greater equity and justice. The three basic principles are that it must promote active citizenship, which means that it empowers learners to exercise their right to political participation (individually and collectively); be contextualised, that is tailored to local realities taking into account the diverse needs of boys and girls in different cultural contexts, including the most marginalised; and be gender-just. Developing quality education is also about targeting the teachers and school management – with well-trained teachers and (female) head teachers, (girl) students have a much higher chance of succeeding in their studies.

Gender just education means that its curriculum includes awareness-raising about gender inequality. It questions beliefs and values about boys and girls, men and women and their roles and diverse identities in society. In school, girls and boys can be educated about their reproductive and sexual rights and receive life-saving information about sexuality and STDs, including HIV and AIDS. This is necessary because worldwide 45% of HIV transmission happens among young people (15-24) and in Africa girls and young women account for 75% of HIV infections among the youth (UNAIDS IATT, 2008). Consciousness about gender discrimination, knowledge of the body, self-esteem and sexuality are extremely important, and when taught well can empower children and young people to have a say over their own bodies and respect the rights and bodies of others. Transformative sexuality education gives learners a positive view of and attitude to sexuality, as well as providing them with information and skills about taking care of their sexual health. Young people who receive this kind of sexuality education are more likely to delay initiating sex and to use protection in the right way when they do have sex (Ibid).

Equally important are the knowledge, skills, attitudes and meaningful participation and empowerment of teachers, especially female teachers. The presence of gender-sensitive teachers and women teachers who apply a rights-based approach that challenges gender stereotypes is vital. Improving the competencies in this regard, introducing participatory styles of learning and involving youth and the development of new, transformative curricula, is important and will be beneficial for students. It also leads to a better professional status and improved morale among women teachers, which makes them more valued in the communities and seen as role models for other women and girls. Another measure could be the increase of female head teachers (which is shockingly low throughout Africa, the Middle East and South and West Asia). They are proven to be more responsive to the needs of girls, promote safer learning environments and liable to stimulate more community involvement, especially in encouraging mothers to become involved within the school.

Quality education has also to do with the number of girls accessing school and how many complete their studies. Seventy-two million primary school-age children, the majority of them being girls, still do not have access to school (UNESCO, 2010). In sub-Saharan Africa, South and West Asia, and in many Arab states (especially in rural areas) the number of girls in the classroom decreases the higher the grade level becomes. The result is that by secondary school the percentage of girls in the classrooms is very low to non-existent. In Sub-Saharan Africa it is reported that many girls of secondary school age can be found in primary schools and do not make it to secondary level (Lloyd, 2009). In the majority of the South 30% of young adults have less than four years of education and this number rises to 50% in eleven countries in sub-Saharan Africa (UNESCO, 2010). Although progress is being made on adult literacy, 759 million adults still lack literacy skills today; two-thirds of them are women (ibid, p. 95). Illiteracy leads to more problems with regard to gender equality, sexuality and the prevention of HIV. For example, when people cannot read it becomes difficult to access and understand the judicial and health systems, or read materials that explain human rights and safety precautions (like why and how to use condoms). It has also been proven that the incidence of GBV decreases when women and girls receive more and better education.

Safe schools, where girls can study free from harassment and abuse, is imperative for quality education (Plan International, 2008). Many girls and boys drop out of school as a result of sexual abuse, corporal punishment, poverty and HIV and AIDS (or even for reasons like not having sanitary napkins for when they are menstruating). While boys usually suffer more violent - and possibly deadly - corporal punishment at the hands of their teachers than their female classmates, sexual harassment and exploitation appear to be overwhelmingly carried out against girls. Girls are vulnerable to attacks not only from teachers and other care-givers, but also from male students, either at school or on the journey to or from school. Social norms that encourage male aggression and female passivity are seen to encourage various forms of violence against girls. Poverty also facilitates the abuse because children are increasingly responsible for the economic welfare of their families. Moreover, teachers are often underpaid, or not paid at all, with some seeing sexual favours from students as 'compensation' (ibid).

Education is not only about the formal classroom. It is just as important to target out of school youth. Throughout the South the majority of the population is under the age of 20, yet the youth seem to be a marginalised group in communities and are not allowed to have a strong voice. Even with projects that involve the youth they are rarely consulted on the process of developing and/or the management of the projects. It is important not only to target the youth but also to involve them as an integral stakeholder in the process. An alliance of organisations in southern Africa and Stop AIDS Now (Hear our Voices! 2009) explain in a study what they noticed were the benefits to their organisation once they involved the youth. They list the following: new ideas and different ways of doing things; information about young people's needs and interests leading to better decision-making; feedback about the effectiveness of existing services to young people and peer-to-peer outreach efforts.

In Nigeria the Girl Power Initiative (GPI), which is also an Innovation Fund recipient, incorporates youth into their organisation by hiring graduates of their youth clubs to be peer educators and some are then trained to be programme staff. How they have built in the triangle of the Fund is by having after-school girl clubs where girls are taught to have confidence in themselves and about their bodies. Dorcas, aged 13, who attends the GPI clubs, explains that at the first GPI sexuality course she was embarrassed when the facilitator mentioned the word sexuality.

> I wanted to leave the class but I could not because the facilitator would notice. I am glad I stayed to the end because I learned the true meaning of the word. I thought the word was for married and elderly people. Now I know it is for all human beings and it teaches us to grow up and be healthy. I told my friend all the things I learned about menstruation and she went to tell her mother who asked her to also attend GPI lessons (GPI, 2009).

Educating young girls on issues concerning gender equity, sexuality and how to prevent HIV as well as building up their confidence is an investment in the development of future Nigerian women leaders. One principal in a school that has a GPI club explains that all the class prefects happen to be part of GPI. This is due to the confidence and communication skills that the GPI clubs build in young women.

Less HIV and AIDS prevalence
Good quality education and more gender equality will help prevent the spread of HIV. It is well known that gender inequality patterns and beliefs lead to different types of GBV such as rape and forced marriages at a young age, FGM, social exclusion and intimidation of HIV positive women, women trafficking, etc. With these types of violence, some of them deeply rooted in cultural traditions, women are more vulnerable to HIV infection than men. Physically and biologically women are more susceptible to HIV because men's semen contains a high concentration of the virus to which the nature of the vagina is receptive: it exposes more skin to potential infection and it is easily torn when violent and forced sex occurs. In unprotected heterosexual intercourse women are twice as likely as men to acquire HIV from an infected partner. This is demonstrated by the 'feminisation' of the HIV and AIDS pandemic: in sub-Saharan Africa almost 57% of HIV infections happen among women and girls (UNAIDS, 2007).
Other cultural practices such as 'dry sex', which is a widespread habit in southern Africa because of the assumption that men enjoy sex more this way, are also dangerous and cause HIV infections. This custom has to do with the idea that women are supposed to be submissive to male pleasure in sexual matters and do not have a say about their own sexual pleasure. Another astonishing practice is the rape of virgins, young girls and children under 12. It is a phenomenon that is driven by beliefs of 'purity' and the hunt for a cure for AIDS.

Furthermore studies from Botswana, Namibia, South Africa, Tanzania and Zimbabwe, show that women who are beaten by their husbands or boyfriends, or are emotionally/financially dominated by their partners, are more likely to be infected than those who live in non-violent households. In India almost 90% of the HIV-positive women interviewed were infected by their husbands while simultaneously blamed for their husbands' illnesses. Women who have been abused and are HIV positive have complex issues to deal with: increased violence, blaming and shaming, forced sterilisation and property grabbing. They are also faced with stigmatisation and subsequent isolation due to being both abused and HIV positive (Oxfam America, 2005: 8-9).

It is mostly the women and girls who bear the biggest burden of care-work when HIV hits their families. This is an important cause of young girls in sub-Saharan Africa dropping out of school. Ensuring access to essential publicly supported services is therefore central to fighting HIV and AIDS, by providing women with good healthcare, quality education, alternative livelihood strategies and tools for protection (ibid: 7).
It is almost needless to say that secondary schooling significantly reduces girls' vulnerability to HIV, since those years of schooling boost the skills and opportunities they need to achieve greater economic independence. At the same time education (formal/informal) is a 'social vaccine' that could contribute to the prevention of further transmission of HIV and therefore prevent increased poverty, gender inequality, rights violation and reduced food and income security.

HIV and issues around gender equality and sexual rights are not always easy topics to address. The Innovation Fund project *Learning about Living* by One World UK and Butterfly Works in Nigeria encourages people to text in questions about sex and HIV and have quick responses texted back by trained professionals. Uju Ofomata, Project Director of the Mobile4Good within the Learning about Living project explains:

Using tools young people are fascinated with such as mobile phones has proven to be effective in increasing their access to sexual reproductive health information. This empowers them to make informed decisions about their sexual health thereby improving health outcomes. Mobile phones and other ICT tools preserve their anonymity and allow them to get accurate information on their own terms, in an environment they are comfortable with, when they need it (Ofomata, 2009).

Innovative computer programming can also be a fun way for young boys and girls to learn how to use a computer and learn more in other subject areas such as reading, spelling and HIV prevention. The Learning about Living project mentioned above (that is now also being piloted in Senegal) also uses interactive computer programming to teach the youth about HIV and gender justice in a way that allows them to learn and ask questions without the concern of being embarrassed to ask in front of their class. It also enables teachers to use interactive ways of teaching about HIV without feeling discomfort when it comes to issues concerning sexuality. One of the lessons learned however from this project is that parents did not feel included in this project and were concerned about the material that their children were being exposed to. This lesson is being incorporated in the future of this project by having more outreach sessions with parents about what their children are learning in school with the computer programmes on SRHR.

The culture link
The Innovation Fund triangle is encircled by 'culture' (see figure 1.). ON embraces the definition of 'culture' as formulated by UNESCO which is "the set of distinctive spiritual, material, intellectual and emotional features of society or a social group, that encompasses, not only art and literature, but lifestyles, ways of living together, value systems, traditions and beliefs" (UNESCO, 2001). It is well known that culture is, has always been and will always be susceptible to change. Striving for more gender justice and less HIV and AIDS infected people is about change: of lifestyles, values systems, traditions and beliefs, in other words: culture. Education plays a big role in this. Moreover, educational systems and the contents of education are shaped by women and men who are also influenced by customs and the spirit of the age. This implies that discriminative and bad quality education can be improved for the better.

How this can be done has to be determined in the best possible way in every cultural and social context. Addressing harmful aspects of culture, celebrating positive ones and working within specific cultural premises are extremely important when planning projects around the triangle of education, gender and HIV. This includes taking into consideration specific aspects of culture or sub-cultures, like the colonial past of certain countries, gay or youth culture, masculinities (working with men) and religion.

Religious contexts, for example, can have a major impact on projects trying to promote gender justice and/or discussions around sexuality and HIV prevention. In fundamental Christian and Muslim communities the discussion of sex and gender justice is sometimes taboo. The use of condoms in the contexts of the two religions can be forbidden. Therefore, to ignore the religious environment when planning a project around these delicate themes can have adverse or even disastrous results. In the example given of GECPD in Somalia, finding the support of religious leaders in the work on the education of people in areas of sexuality and HIV is an important part of the project.

Another example is found in an external evaluation of the Innovation Fund partners in India (Resource centre for gender & education, 2009). It was discovered that there was a high degree of nervousness about the issues of homosexuality within the peer educators of many of the different projects. Although homosexuality and transgender is common in these cultures it is seen as something that cannot be discussed. This makes it a difficult undertaking to make sure that all the messages are free from homophobia, fear and prejudices. These culturally-difficult topics can be complex to broach but it is an important lesson for the project organisers and Oxfam Novib just how important it is for the trainers to be well trained and have cohesion about messaging that will not increase stigma, fears and discrimination.

'Culture' has another connotation in the sense of dance, theatre, music, humour, art and more. These entertaining and artistic forms can be excellent ways and powerful tools for teaching people about HIV and broader issues of SRHR, issues that they might have previously been closed to because of taboos. In Tanzania, the Innovation Fund partner Yaden uses theatre to educate communities on issues from teen pregnancy to HIV. One audience member explained that she was moved to tears when one of the actors explained that the story was based on her own life of being kicked out of her home after she was discovered to be pregnant and she vowed that she would start an open dialogue with her daughter about sexuality. See also textbox below for an example from Bangladesh.

Conclusions
From the foregoing it is clear that ON believes that value systems, traditions and (sub)-cultural beliefs and practices have a major impact when looking at gender inequality patterns, the quality and contents of education and the prevalence of HIV and AIDS. Patriarchal cultures heavily affect girls and women's position in society, resulting in subordination, discrimination and women/femininity being less valued. When women have such an inferior status, it affects, for example, the choices that parents make in regards to choosing their boy children over their girl children to attend school and it is directly linked to having less power to demand condoms or refuse sex. As stated before, biologically, women are more susceptible to HIV infection. Cultural customs like FGM, 'dry sex' and early marriages increase the risk and also make women suffer more once they are infected. Education (formal or informal) is one of the motors for changing these practices or beliefs.

Although the gathering of the results and lessons learned from the Innovation Fund projects is still an ongoing process, as projects are still in the final phases and the feedback and evaluations are still underway, at this moment we can say that the focus of the triangle has resulted in interesting lessons and new innovative methods of working. This was shown when experiences were shared, organisations were linked and an organisational memory was kept at the Cross-cultural Learning Conference in South Africa about interventions that address HIV and AIDS, sexuality, gender and education (SAfAIDS, Oxfam Novib and Hivos et al, 2010). This should result in building and shaping stronger projects in the future.

One issue that emerged during the conference in South Africa in April 2010 on the topic of "Education, gender and HIV in a cross cultural perspective" that involved many Innovation

Fund partners, is that organisations are struggling with how to measure behavioural changes.[4] This is an area that ON would like to concentrate further on in the future, as it is essential to presenting the work and objectives that we and our partners are trying to do and achieve.

> **Multimedia in the prevention of HIV and promotion of gender justice**
> Information provided by Rashida Parveen, Senior Manager, Adolescent Development Programme, BRAC, Bangladesh
>
> In Bangladesh, the Innovation Fund supported a BRAC project where they showed films in small villages to start the discussion on HIV. One drama focused on prevention and contamination information on HIV and AIDS. The second one focused more on societal acceptance and positive attitude towards a HIV and AIDS positive person. Over 250 shows were arranged. Two posters on HIV and AIDS also focusing on adolescents were designed and developed. "We would like to test our blood, can BRAC help us to do that?" said a young woman of Hilli village in Jamalpur after watching the drama on HIV and AIDS in multi-media.
>
> Using audio-visual material in the remotest areas of the country was a new approach that received a very positive response from the communities. In the villages, entertainment options are limited; therefore, this initiative was able to reach the wider community. Thousands of people attended each of the shows. Two dramas on the HIV and AIDS theme and a drama on gender, child marriage and dowry were also developed and shown.
>
> The project also involved working with 8,715 adolescent clubs throughout the country that looked at the issues around the themes of gender justice, HIV and education. What BRAC has discovered and what they are proud about in this project is the significant impact on rural adolescents in Bangladesh in terms of their awareness-building regarding social issues. Parents' attitudes towards gender equality have improved significantly due to programme intervention. It has also been found that adolescents' access to healthcare centres has increased significantly due to programme participation; and the awareness regarding gender equality both in family and professional life has also improved. Adolescent as well as community awareness regarding HIV and AIDS and of the consequences of taking drug substances has also increased as a result of programme participation.
>
> Involvement of community people before the project started was a significant reason for the success of the project. In every village of the project area, a village committee was formed to work towards achieving the goal of the project.

---

[4] See chapter on monitoring and evaluating.

Changing the River's Flow in Senegal
Information provided by Adama Mbengue from FAWE Senegal and Cheikhou Toure from Enda Graf Sahel

In Senegal the organisations Enda Graf Sahel and FAWE Senegal work together on a project funded by the Innovation Fund. Enda Graf is an organisation that has been working on alternative education with generations of children that were not able to attend formal school in a programme they called "école de la Rue" (*school of the road*). FAWE is a prominent, Africa-wide forum with connections across social strata and a mandate to address the gender gap in education.

The programme they developed is aimed above all at the people falling outside the regular public education system. It provides methodological support to local organisations, based on three concepts: gender, participatory democracy, and sexual reproductive health rights (SRHR).

These three concepts lead to the final goal of reducing inequalities and injustice, by means of offering alternative educational methods via local organisations. Each of the 30 participating local structures submits a plan for support and funding around one or more axes. The programme strengthens individual organisations on the one hand, and promotes networking among organisations on the other, to jointly lobby by influencing national (political) decision-making around education.

Some of the innovations within the project are working with the Koranic schools to modernise their curriculum and making it more gender-sensitive and including SRHR. Other innovations include working with the informal education systems and training trainers in the approach called *Tuseme* (a Kiswahili world which means 'To speak without embarrassment'). This programme works with children to understand and resolve the problems they are facing academically and socially.

FAWEU girl-child education: A strategy in promoting gender equity, HIV and AIDS awareness and breaking cultural barriers in Uganda
*Special Note. This project is only partially funded by the Innovation Fund
Information provided by Josephine Pedun, Programme Officer, FAWE Uganda chapter

Girls' education in sub-Saharan Africa, particularly in Uganda, continues to be plagued by a variety of socio-cultural and economic barriers. In Uganda, the implementation of the Universal Primary Education (UPE) programme in 1997 has resulted in increased access to education from over 2.5 million to 7.5 million in 2008. This has consequently narrowed the gender gap in primary schools to about 1% (51% boys and 49% girls). Likewise the gender gap in secondary schools has reduced as the absolute number of girls enrolled in the first year of secondary level also increased by 30,231 (31%) from 98,392 (FY 2006/07) to 128,623 (FY 2007/08) i.e. the ratio improving from 45:55 to 46:54. (MoE 2008).

Remarkable achievements have also been realised in reducing the HIV and AIDS prevalence rate down from more than 20% in 1980s to about 6% by the year 2000. However, the HIV and AIDS levels have stagnated since then, showing marginal increase in prevalence over the past few years. (UNAIDS/WHO 2008)

Despite the achievements, other barriers exist but none more pronounced than culture, which remains one of the barriers in the fight against HIV and AIDS and in the attainment of gender equity in education. Many girls in Uganda are married off young, while some are defiled because of the prevailing cultural belief that sex with virgins cures HIV and AIDS. According to various reports, there are increasing cases of defilement currently estimated at 57% (ANNPPCAN Uganda 2009) exposing girls to high risk of HIV and AIDS. Other reports by the Uganda Demographic Health Survey (DHS EdData Survey 2001) indicated that early marriage or pregnancy is an important factor for girls aged 13-18 years dropping out of primary school. Pre-marital pregnancy among girls is stigmatised both in school and in most African communities mainly on moralistic grounds, without addressing factors that lead to pregnancy among schoolgirls.

A recent study conducted in the Karamoja a region in northern Uganda by FAWEU (FAWEU 2009) indicates that girls perform poorly at school because of distractions from concentrating on studies, such as domestic chores, entertainments, allurements from men for sex, pressure from parents to get married early, sexual advancements from boys, all worsened by the fact that they are enrolled in school late when they are perceived as old and ready to be wives. The study further revealed that retention of girls in school among the Pokot in Karamoja is low mainly because of FGM, which is a strong tradition. Girls between the ages of 11-14 are supposed to go through the practice and are married off almost immediately after initiation. These cultural practices (such as early marriages etc), among other factors, have reinforced GBV within the school and home environments.

A number of studies done to explore the relationship between poverty, gender and education in the country (UNICEF 1999, GoU 1999, MoES, 1995) describe the ways in which girls are found to be disadvantaged in relation to boys. Poverty, combined with discriminative cultural attitudes, often serves to worsen already existing gender biases. When schooling costs become a pertinent issue and a choice has to be made between sending a boy or girl to school, the boy is usually given precedence. This choice is driven by societal construction of gender where male children are expected to carry on the family tree across generations and are therefore accorded more value than female children. Perceived returns to parents of educating their daughters beyond primary school tend to be lower than for their sons, particularly in patrilocal systems where girls join their husbands. Reluctance to educate girls for the other family into which they are expected to marry is compounded by the opportunity costs which continue to get higher for poor households who depend considerably on the labour of their children in order to supplement household income and help to take care of the sick, especially in this era of HIV and AIDS. Early marriage, especially in the case of girls, is a strategy commonly used by poor families to raise income for the rest of household members, and is more practised in rural than urban areas. Many girls perceive marriage as an escape route from family poverty, while the common cultural practice of charging bride wealth brings quick and substantial income to her family.

Although Uganda has registered progress in terms of access to HIV and AIDS treatment for both men and women, the figure is probably lower for women and girls because of gender-based barriers such as stigma, discrimination and violence. In many communities HIV positive girls are more severely discriminated as they are seen as prostitutes. In many cases they suffer stigma in school, which limits the achievement of gender equality in education. The HIV and AIDS pandemic has caused an increase in the school dropout rates, reinforcing wider problems arising from poverty and social discrimination such as orphanhood and stigmatisation.

Today FAWEU has documented good practices in promotion of girls' education that have been replicated in other regions in Uganda. FAWEU participates in formulation of gender-related policies in a bid to close the gender gap in education. FAWEU's demonstrable interventions include: the sexual maturation management that equips young girls to better manage menstruation. This is because studies have indicated that poor management of menstruation is, among others, a major cause of dropout. The programme also empowers girls and boys with life skills to better understand their sexuality and to promote responsible behaviour. The aim is to provide young people with adequate knowledge on sexual reproductive health in order to reduce unprotected sex, unintended pregnancy, drug abuse, unsafe abortion, and sexually transmitted infections, including HIV. FAWEU emphasis is on engaging key stakeholders at the community level, encouraging, especially, the cultural and religious leaders to take the lead in sensitising the public to promote girls education and to abolish harmful traditional practices against girls and women like FGM.

FAWEU has the Gender Responsive Programme that equips teachers with knowledge, skills and appreciation of gender-responsive teaching methodologies, understanding of gender and related concepts and understanding of a gender-responsive school. The programme has come up with a Centre of Excellence/Gender-Responsive School initiative that not only makes the school child-friendly but also takes care of the girl-children environmentally, socially and physically. Girls' education clubs *TUSEME* (Lets Speak) have been introduced in schools where the students share various life skills to run and manage their daily life and cope with challenges.

FAWEU provides scholarships to girls from poor households who perform well at National Primary Leaving Examinations but fail to join secondary school because their parents or guardians cannot afford the monetary costs involved or force girls to marry. This started as a small effort, but because it was managed effectively and efficiently, the project attracted large funds from donor agencies and now over 4,000 girls have benefited from the scholarship at secondary school level. In addition, FAWEU promotes science studies by empowerment of girls to know that they can also compete with boys in sciences through the use of role models to inspire the girls into taking on sciences. These programmes by FAWEU aim to equip girls and women with adequate skills and knowledge to effectively compete on the job market, and execute their roles through strategic projects that address exclusion and deprivation of girls and women from education.

FAWEU's achievements would not have been possible, given the complexity of factors behind gender inequity and inequalities in education, without the programmatic, intellectual and resource-based inputs from its various partners. To FAWEU, girl-child education remains the main strategy in promoting gender equity, HIV and AIDS awareness and breaking cultural barriers in Uganda.

References

Antrobus, Peggy. "The Global Women's Movement: Origins, Issues and Strategies." London-New York: Zed Books, 2004.

Goetz, Anne Marie. "Gender Justice, Citizenship and Entitlements: Core Concepts, Central Debates and New Directions for Research." In: *Gender Justice, Citizenship and Development*. Mukhopadhyay, Maitrayee and Navsharan Singh (eds). New Delhi: Zubaan, an imprint of Kali for Women, 2007, p. 15-58.

GPI (Girls' Power Initiative). "Girls Power through education." External Evaluation, GPI, 2009.

Lloyd, C. "New lessons: The power of educating adolescent girls." Population Council, 2009, p. 1.

Ofomata, Uju. Interview. June 2010.

Ostergaard, Lisa. "Género y Desarrollo, Guía práctica." In: *Serie Documentos del Instituto de la Mujer*. Madrid, 11 (1991). Translated from Spanish into English and adapted by the authors.

Oxfam America. "AIDS and Gender Inequalities in Southern Africa: A Rights-based Perspective." 2005.

Plan International. "Learn Without Fear". 2008.

Resource centre for gender & education. "Mainphase Evaluation." Delhi, 2009.

Restrepo Ramirez, Dalia. "Los derechos socio-culturales y sus implicaciones para la Socializacion y otros contextos." In: *Documentos de Familia Manizales*, Universidad de Caldas 5 (1992).

SAfAIDS, Oxfam Novib and Hivos, et al.. "HIV/Culture Confluence." Conference, Johannesburg, South Africa, 2010, April 12 to 15.

UNAIDS (Joint United Nations Programme on HIV/AIDS) "2007 AIDS Epidemic Update" Geneva, Switzerland: UNAIDS, 2007.

UNAIDS IATT. "Girls Education and HIV Prevention". 2008: http://unesdoc.unesco.org/images/0015/001586/158670e.pdf

UNESCO. "UNESCO Universal Declaration on Cultural Diversity." Paris: UNESCO, 2001.

UNESCO. "Global Monitoring Report on Education For All." Oxford University Press, 2010.

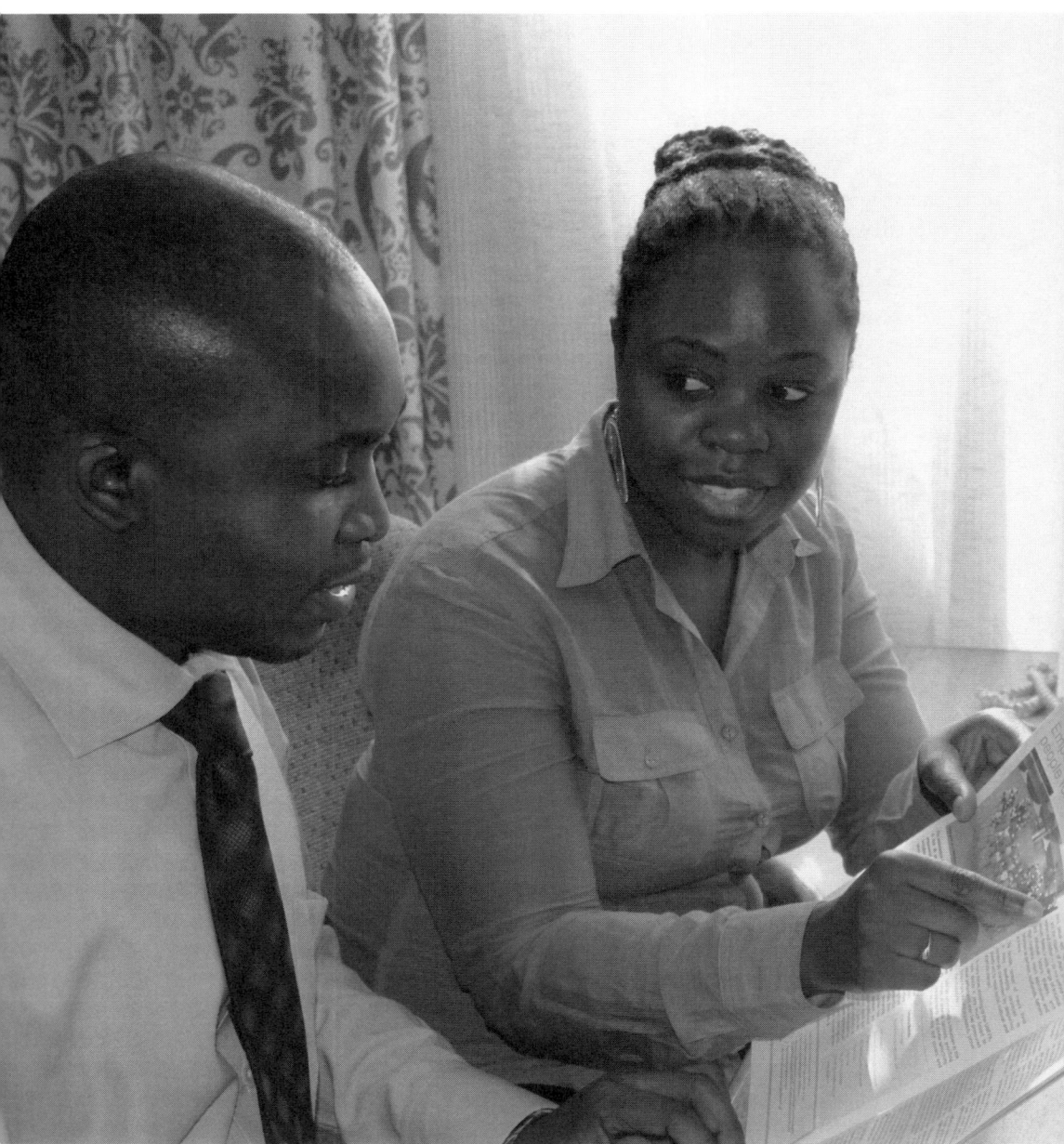

Communicating HIV and AIDS, sexuality and gender messages across cultures: The place of a newsletter in an Internet era

Eliezer F. Wangulu

In broad readership studies, non-governmental organisations (NGOs) tend to be passive when it comes to information and communication, management and distribution. Some of them lack effective communication strategies to tackle the ever-changing reproductive health scenario. Many organisations working in the social development sector do not have a communications strategy in place, nor have they committed staff and personnel to manage or document their programming efforts.

When organisations are just getting started, their leaders can often prize themselves on not being burdened with what seems to be bureaucratic overhead, that is, as extensive written policies and procedures. Writing something down can be seen as a sign of bureaucracy and thus to be avoided. As the organisation grows, it needs more communication and feedback to remain healthy (McNamara, 2010). Some perceive establishing a communications department or engaging a communications officer as an unnecessary overhead. Prudent managers should always recognise the need for increased, reliable communications both internally and with external stakeholders.

Yet information and communication are powerful tools for AIDS service organisations (ASOs), human rights advocates, and people living with HIV (PLHIV) organisations, which use information and communication to enable advocacy, mobilisation, networking, and capacity-building. Information and communication play critical roles in addressing some of the political factors that limit effective responses, by facilitating greater transparency and monitoring of government through civil society and mass media reporting, and by encouraging increased democratic participation. Information and communication offer valuable tools to hold countries to their political and legal commitments to HIV and AIDS, expressed internationally, regionally, and nationally (OEDC, 2001).

The power of the media cannot be underestimated, for information can confer the capacity to act appropriately, whether by protecting oneself from infection or taking steps to influence decision -makers. Information is the source of considerable personal and social power, and has the capacity to shift some of the power differentials at the heart of the epidemic.

The African AIDS epidemic continues to pose severe public health and developmental problems for many African nations. A primary impediment in the fight against AIDS is a lack of information and communication about the disease. Information and communication, as well as information and communication technologies (ICT), hold vast potential to hinder the spread of the disease, as key elements of all aspects of HIV and AIDS strategies, including prevention, treatment and care and protection of human rights. They offer potential solutions to misinformation and myths, silence and denial, and stigma and discrimination against people living with HIV and AIDS (ibid).

Household or individual income is an important determinant of the presence of PCs and the extent of Internet access in homes. Income distribution is particularly important early in the diffusion of new technology, with higher income groups acquiring ICTs early and leading uptake (ibid). In Africa, where the mobile phone is clearly dominating, fixed telephone lines remain the exception and penetration is at three per 100 inhabitants, by far the lowest in the world. The limited availability of fixed lines has also been a barrier to the uptake of fixed broadband and it is most likely that Africa's broadband market will be dominated by mobile broadband. The International Telecommunications Union (ITU) started collecting data on mobile broadband subscribers in 2005 and data show that while uptake is on the rise, the rollout of mobile broadband services is concentrated in the developed world (ITU, 2010).

This trend has, doubtlessly, been replicated in Africa and other developing countries where penetration has been generally very slow, but mainly in homes due to low individual incomes. Unfortunately, regions with the high levels of poverty in the world, especially the sub-Saharan Africa, are the worst affected by the HIV pandemic.

This chapter seeks to share experiences on how the Royal Tropical Institute (KIT) has been using *Exchange on HIV and AIDS, Sexuality and Gender,* a quarterly magazine it publishes jointly with Southern Africa HIV and AIDS Information Dissemination (SAfAIDS) based in Pretoria, to empower its target readership in the global South for improved programming. The question this chapter seeks to respond to is whether the dawn of e-publishing has spelt doom for publications such as *Exchange on HIV and AIDS, Sexuality and Gender* that seek to empower their readerships across differrent cultural settings in the global South.

Tom Wilson, Professor at the Department of Information Studies, University of Sheffield in the UK, in an essay titled *Electronic publishing and the future of the book*, states that the aims of those publishing electronically may be very much the same as those publishing in book form adding that one needs only to scan the World Wide Web for a short time to discover this fact. Just like the printed versions, electronic publishing, he adds, has pages of humour as well as pages of information.

According to Professor Wilson, electronic publishing has very specific non-book characteristics that distinguish it from print publication. Their ability to be produced and disseminated very rapidly - once a page of text has been coded with HTML tags it can be published immediately - the book takes much longer to produce and distribute; text can be updated or corrected with the same immediacy, whereas a book must either go through a second edition, or, if the error is caught in time, have an erratum slip inserted; electronic publications can be disseminated world-wide without the need for separate rights negotiations for different countries and without the costs of distribution or reprinting; where an electronic publication is charged for, the producer does not incur the costs associated with retail bookselling, that is, there are no "middleman" costs.

Some of the disadvantages he cites regarding e-publishing include the demand for access to relatively advanced technology on the part of both the producer and the consumer of information or entertainment - even the base level of provision is still expensive for the ordinary citizen; mobile computers, notebooks and smaller, are either too big or have screens that are too small, or are otherwise inadequate for use across the full range of environments in which a book can be read; the technology is still, to a significant degree, user-unfriendly to many people; the technology consumes a greater amount of energy in its use than the book (Wilson, 1997).

Exchange on HIV and AIDS, Sexuality and Gender

Over the years, *Exchange on HIV and AIDS, Sexuality and Gender* magazine has been published in English, French, Portuguese and Spanish enabling a good number of target readers in the Global South to share their experiences in the implementation of HIV and AIDS, sexuality and gender projects and programmes. The French and Spanish versions are no longer published due to funding problems. The *Exchange* plays, in a small way, a strategic role in bridging the digital divide through promoting networking and information to inform projects and programme implementation for organisations. The key objective of the publication is to share information, good practices and experiences regarding HIV and AIDS, sexuality and gender work among organisations and countries, mainly in the global South, for improved programming.

Most of the magazine's hard copies are distributed in sub-Saharan Africa. In this region, a large share of the magazine is distributed by SAfAIDS in southern Africa, the region that bears the heaviest burden of HIV and AIDS. Lately, there has been increased demand for the magazine in the region. As a result, KIT and SAfAIDS are seeking to increase the production of the hard copies of the magazine to meet this demand.

Background to the *Exchange* magazine

The magazine was established in 1988 under the title *AIDS Health Promotion Exchange* as a joint effort between KIT and the World Health Organisation (WHO). The partnership with SAfAIDS began in 1995, and with it came the change of the magazine's name to *AIDS/STD Health Promotion Exchange*. In 1998, the magazines' name again changed to *Sexual Health Exchange*. In 2005, it switched its title again, settling for the current *Exchange on HIV and AIDS, Sexuality and Gender* to respond to the increasing demands of the evolving pandemic.

The magazine is currently published in English and Portuguese. The Portuguese version is titled *Intercambio*. The aim of the magazine in terms of its editorial content is to highlight HIV, AIDS, and sexuality and gender issues relevant to Africa, the Caribbean, Latin America and South East Asia. There are cases where articles which are educative or informative, but from outside the above regions, are carried in the magazine.

The mission of the *Exchange* magazine

The publication's mission is to facilitate the international exchange of experiences and information on HIV prevention and sexual health promotion in developing countries. By carrying out this mission the publishers aim to contribute to professional development of personnel involved in HIV and AIDS, sexuality and gender work in developing countries and countries in transition so that they can improve their interventions, products and outcomes.

Target audience
The exchange has primary and secondary readership. The primary target includes professionals in HIV and AIDS and sexual and reproductive health programmes and services, working at local and national levels in developing countries and countries in transition, e.g. programme managers, health and HIV and AIDS educators, community health workers, social workers, nurses, doctors working in NGOs, FBOs, CBOs or health facilities. On the other hand, secondary readers of the magazine include policy makers and programme managers in governmental institutions; INGOs; UN agencies; media personnel; librarians or personnel in AIDS Resource Centres and libraries; researchers, teachers and trainers.

Regional representation
Africa, the Caribbean, Latin America and South East Asia are represented on the publication's production team by editorial advisors who are experts in the areas of HIV and AIDS, sexuality and gender and they advise the Managing Editor on topical issues peculiar to their regions that require to be highlighted in the magazine. Selecting themes to be covered by the publication is mainly an activity for KIT and SAfAIDS and also in consultation with editorial advisors. Once themes have been identified, the Managing Editor sends out calls for articles through various e-fora; KIT and SAfAIDS websites; through the magazine itself and sometimes organisations may be contacted and requested to submit an article on the basis of their being involved in programmes or projects relevant to the theme. KIT and SAfAIDS organise an annual meeting where themes for subsequent editions are identified.

Themes that have been carried by the magazine in recent times include: Minority sexual practices and how they contribute to HIV infection; Psychological, gender, cultural and sexual behavioural implications of male circumcision as a method of HIV prevention; How multiple and concurrent sexual relationships accelerate HIV infections; Cross-cultural learning on HIV, AIDS, sexuality, gender and education; Male reproductive health in the context of HIV prevention and How intergenerational sex contributes to HIV infections. The publications' (*Exchange and Intercambio*) articles are mainly short and written in easy-to-read, non-scholarly language on themes relevant to their readers.

Print run and dissemination
The print run for the *Exchange* is 3,000 copies per edition while that of *Intercambio* is 1,000. The bulk of these issues, about two thirds, are delivered to the SAfAIDS Country Office in Harare, Zimbabwe for further distribution to partner organisations in southern Africa. Some readers also access the magazines electronically. The magazines are available on KIT and SAfAIDS websites and can be downloaded in portable document format (PDF) (www.exchange-magazine.info). During the fourth quarter of 2009, *Exchange* recorded 11,123 downloads.

Separate PDFs for all articles can be found on the OAI-PMH compliant repository, Search4Dev and consequently accessible through harvesting information services around the world. SAfAIDS distributes the *Exchange* and *Intercambio* through a database of their contacts in southern Africa. *Exchange* is also distributed in Eastern Africa and West Africa while *Intercambio* is only sent to readers in Portuguese-speaking Angola and Mozambique. Currently, *Exchange* and *Intercambio* are two of the few international magazines that are printed and distributed freely in developing countries.

Why hard copies

According to an article titled *Africa joins the Internet bandwagon* carried online by *Africa Business Pages* (http://www.africa-business.com/features/internet.html -accessed July 9, 2010), at least 45 of the 54 capital cities in Africa in 2009 offered their residents live public Internet access services and of these eight countries have local dial-up access throughout their more rural regions. The article further stated that rapid adaptation of the Internet as a business tool over the past three years was the main reason for the surge in connections, but over-regulation and poor telecommunication infrastructure continued to pose serious obstacles to true cyber-connectivity.

According to the New Partnership for Africa's Development (NEPAD), the reasons for the African digital divide are diverse. According to the pan-African organisation, poor ICT infrastructure, combined with weak policy and regulatory frameworks and limited human resources, has resulted in inadequate access to affordable telephones, broadcasting, computers and the Internet.[5]

The NEPAD report further states that there are encouraging trends of growth in Internet usage, with rapid growth in most urban areas in Africa, and current availability in every capital city. However, the vast majority of Internet subscribers are located in Northern Africa and South Africa, with a smattering of subscribers in the remaining forty-nine sub-Saharan African countries (ibid).

In another June 2010 article in the *it news Africa,* authored by Brian Adero (http://www.itnewsafrica.com/?p=8314, accessed August 2, 2010,) the Eassy fibre optic cable which was launched in June 2010 offers a direct route to Europe, and is the largest cable system in sub-Saharan Africa. Eassy landing stations, according to Adero's article, include Port Sudan, Djibouti, Mombasa in Kenya, Dar-es-salaam in Tanzania, Moroni in Comoros Islands, Toliary in Madagascar, Maputo in Mozambique and Mtuzini in South Africa. The 10,000 kilometre cable cost $263 million and has a capacity of 1.4 terabits per second, making it the largest submarine cable system serving the African continent. The article further stated that Eassy will be the first East Coast system to connect on a direct route to Europe, making it the lowest latency system for traffic to key Internet peering points in Europe and North America because other systems use a longer path to reach Europe, through connections in either India or United Arab Emirates (UAE).

Although there is a lot of useful information available on the Internet, studies show that many members of *Exchange* magazine target readership still do not have access or good access to these resources. The digital divide problem is well-known, yet an increasing number of international organisations and publishers have stopped publishing print copies of their various resources. A typical situation is a small non-profit organisation in Africa with only one computer, and, if it is lucky, that computer is connected to the Internet. This one computer happens to be located in the office of the Director.

Many lower cadre staff use free Hotmail and Yahoo accounts and go to Internet cafes to read and write their mail. Downloading and printing PDFs in such environments can be a tedious and expensive affair. Even though connectivity is increasing rapidly, figures provided by the International Telecommunications Union show that, especially in countries with high

HIV prevalence, access to the Internet is still limited. Yet these organisations need the information that would empower them to carry out their mandates effectively. It is against this background that KIT and SAfAIDS continue to produce hard copies of *Exchange* and *Intercambio*.

The subscription policy of the *Exchange* states that there are limited numbers of print copies available for those who have no access to the Internet. The secondary readership category that includes media, trainers, teachers, librarians and information officers are allowed free print subscription, but this is subject to availability. The electronic edition is freely available to anyone. For those who cannot easily download PDFs a low-resolution file can be sent by e-mail.

Readership survey

A readership survey for *Exchange* undertaken in 2009 found that respondents receive the magazine in either hard (paper) or soft (electronic) versions. Few organisations receive the publication in both formats. It became clear that fledgling CBOs and other younger organisations prefer the print version of the magazine, which is easier to use, circulate and share. And not surprisingly, most of those that preferred print copies were from areas facing communication challenges, such as limited access to the Internet, lack of electricity and lack of access to telephones.

The purpose of the readership survey, administered through both online and paper questionnaires, in-depth interviews and focus group discussions, was to find out if and how the magazine contributes to HIV and AIDS-related programmes by providing invaluable information for implementers to improve their approaches and also, if the presentation of the publication was done in a way that is preferred by the target readership. Its outcome would enable the production team of the magazine to make the necessary changes required to meet the specific needs of the target readership in terms of content and presentation.

The survey also served to explore other innovative ways of using the magazine, such as being a focus around which other offshoot activities related to its theme area could be organised. These activities could include conferences, meetings and other fora bringing together participants from different cultural settings to share best practices.

The cultural link

Culture as an instrument of empowerment is born of the belief that culture itself represents the continuum of good, indifferent and bad. The goal of cultural empowerment is to ensure that an intervention is developed with the idea of *not* only the bad in mind, but to also promote the good and recognise the unique or indifferent aspects of culture (Airhihenbuwa and DeWitt, 2004).

Projects addressing HIV, sexuality and gender are implemented in cultural contexts. Similarly, readers of publications interpret the information from a cultural standpoint. This is because culture "…permeates all aspects of life. It contains the local perception of the meaning of life and of what for a local population simply constitutes a 'good life'. It is a matrix, the software of social life, its 'symbolic engine'. It can be a source of positive dynamism. People, in the last analysis, are the repository of local knowledge (Eade, 2002). *Exchange* endeavours to highlight topical HIV and AIDS, sexuality and gender issues from various geographical contexts and a variety of cultural settings in the global South while taking cognisance of the inherent cultural sensitivities of its target readers.

Print versions preferred
The *Exchange* survey also found that the print version of the magazine is preferred, as illustrated by 68 per cent of online responses. However, some respondents preferred to receive both versions to suit their immediate needs. Where readers preferred electronic copies, it was because they found it easier to circulate to fellow staff members or send it via e-mail to their networks. Special articles of interest were 'flagged' and distributed on request. In the case of hard copies, readers found it useful to discuss certain articles through reference, or engage in a 'read and pass on' trend (Stally, Ngwerume and Kimemiah, 2009).

Practical use of the *Exchange* magazine
According to the survey, readers have taken advantage of the *Exchange*'s open policy for use of articles, and they have done this in many ways to enhance their own programme efforts. These include awareness-building, community support and sharing of best practices.

The *Exchange* has played a pivotal role in supporting community outreach activities and promoting gender awareness. For example, the Community Working Group on Health (CWGH) has used information from the magazine to conduct community health education awareness campaigns. It also helps strengthen women's participation in decision-making through empowerment on critical gender issues such as domestic violence. Furthermore, the *Exchange* assists organisations in their efforts to empower communities on pertinent issues in the area of sexual and reproductive health rights issues. Also, it engages the community in dialogue on the topic of sexual networks, extra-marital relationships and HIV risks, which are pertinent to the work of some of the organisations receiving the magazine such as the Batsirai Group in Chinhoyi, Zimbabwe (ibid).

Beyond the specified readership numbers, there is a wider distribution of information. The majority (90%) of readers are more likely to share the articles with others, thereby increasing the knowledge base derived from the publication. Complementary to this is the use of Resource Centres (RCs) and other fora where groups of readers can access the publication. Organisations such as SAfAIDS have multi-disciplinary Resource Centres where the publication is placed alongside other HIV-related material. In this regard, interest groups such as researchers who are not subscribers can refer to the publication for specific purposes. Furthermore, the Zimbabwe AIDS Network (ZAN) distributes the magazine at public events such as the Zimbabwe Agricultural Show, Zimbabwe NGO Expo and the Zimbabwe International Trade Fair (ZITF).

From an academic perspective, the survey found that the magazine provides detailed facts to inform research on its theme areas. According to a researcher with the Institute of Development Studies (IDS), the *Exchange* has been a point of reference when reviewing literature. The results of the survey also show that the magazine has benefited readers in other innovative ways as follows: Source of information to inform drama on HIV and AIDS; to support in-house communication strategies on HIV and AIDS; as a reference point for field facilitators during community discussions on HIV, AIDS, sexuality and gender; for informing project proposal writing; supporting information for health lectures and as content to share in workshops and seminars.

Similar examples also emerged from discussions with informants during the in-depth interviews carried out as part of the readership survey in Zimbabwe. For example, an umbrella of HIV and AIDS organisations serving people living with HIV and AIDS in Zimbabwe (ZNNP+) detailed below how the network had gained practical benefits from this joint KIT-SAfAIDS publication:

> Through the Exchange, ZNNP+ has successfully created a partnership between the Network of Positive Women and the International Community of Women Living with HIV and AIDS (ICW). This partnership was established through information derived from the Links and Resources section of the magazine. As a result, the ZNNP+ provincial coordinator was sponsored to attend a meeting in South Africa through partnerships created with the ICW. Through learning from activities shared through ICW and related meetings, women living with HIV in Zimbabwe have now embarked on a strategy to revive the Network of Positive Women (ibid).

Readers' opinions of the *Exchange*
According to the readership survey report, most readers indicated that the magazine provides useful perspectives of other experts working in the same fields, which was enlightening, and that the editorial content provides fresh aspects of HIV and tackles health issues in a comprehensive manner. Others said that the publication touches on the key areas that affect sexuality and HIV and AIDS, describing it as "an excellent resource tool". A good number of the readership survey respondents indicated that the magazine demystifies sexuality, giving them the information they need when having to deal with similar issues in their contexts.

Challenges facing the publication
Challenges have been noted in terms of translating important information during training sessions that are conducted in the vernacular. A trainer of home-based care (HBC) volunteers with Batsiranai Narini in Zimbabwe indicated that it is difficult to translate some of the technical terms into the local language. According to the respondent, "some of the terms are technical and thus open to diverse interpretations." This is understandable given that in some circumstances, trainees are illiterate or not well-versed in English" (ibid).
In terms of distribution, the bulk of the hard copies of the magazine are sent to organisations in southern Africa by SAfAIDS and currently, there is no mechanism to track the exercise with a view to ascertaining whether the distribution strategy is effective or not. This can be improved by getting the support of an effective and 'live' database for the magazine.

"The magazine is for the elite at present and not many people get access to it at grassroots level" a reader was quoted saying of the publication. What this reader implied was that it was difficult to access the publication and this is understandable because only 3,000 hard copies of *Exchange* are printed. KIT and SAfAIDS have been working jointly to raise more funds to increase the print-run to meet the increased demand of the publication, especially in southern Africa. So far these efforts have not yielded fruit.

Suggestions for improvement
Beyond launching a call for articles there is a need to promote greater involvement of stakeholders through innovative participatory strategies such as poll voting to select future themes; and direct interaction between the editorial team and readers. There is also a need for a feedback mechanism, while some readers have suggested that the publication carry a calendar of key meetings, trainings, events and workshops. Other suggestions include adding more colour to the magazine; using bullet points more to add variety and make it more pleasing to the eye and translating the publication into appropriate vernacular languages, e.g. Kiswahili, and considering distribution at community-level.

Conclusions and recommendations
As argued above, the advent of the Internet has ushered in an era of e-publishing, which is immediate and cheaper. Yet a majority of *Exchange* readers, according to the survey and other findings, still lack access to the Internet or reliable access that would enable them to source relevant information from the Internet that would inform their HIV, AIDS, gender and sexuality interventions. This constituency happens to be in the global South, which coincidentally, is the region most ravaged by HIV and AIDS. This is the target readership that should be catered for through publication of *Exchange* and similar publications. The programme officer working for a small CBO serving the people of an outlying village called Mukangu in Kakamega district of western Kenya who is on the *Exchange* mailing list will need the hard copy version of the publication for some time to come. And similarly so for other readers in such remote locations with poor roads, no electricity and lack of access to the Internet.

To some degree, the objectives of the magazine have been achieved through mainly supporting awareness-building on the magazine's theme areas by its target readership; sharing of best practices from the Global South; supporting community outreach activities and promoting gender-awareness, while also empowering minority groups by echoing their aspirations that fall within the ambit of the magazine's theme areas.

However, to successfully move forward in striving to meet its broader objectives, the production team will need to take on board well-meaning suggestions from its readership base by factoring them into the entire magazine production process so that *Exchange* is a readers' publication. Also, there is an urgent need to revise the distribution strategy to ensure that it is effective and that both print and electronic versions of the magazine reach a good percentage of those who need them.

The above could be partly achieved through coming up with a strategy whereby new partnerships or old ones are consolidated or activated to widen the distribution channels. This could also entail creating links with focal points in key strategic organisations such as information and/or communications officers to oversee the distribution of *Exchange* in their organisations.

References

Adero, Brian. "IT news Africa." accessed 2 August 2010:
   http://www.itnewsafrica.com/?p=8314

Airhihenbuwa C. O. and J. DeWitt. "Culture and African contexts of HIV/AIDS prevention, care and support." In: Webster: Journal of Social Aspects of HIV/AIDS Research Alliance. 1(2004) 1 May.

Eade, D. (ed.). "Development and culture: A development in practice reader." Oxfam in association with Word Faiths Development Dialogue. 2002.

ITU. "Global ICT Developments" accessed 25 August 2010:
   http://www.itu.int/ITU-D/ict/statistics/ict/index.html

McNamara, Carter. "Basics in Internal Organizational Communications." Adapted from: Field Guide to Leadership and Supervision, accessed 25 August 2010:
   http://managementhelp.org/mrktng/org_cmm.htm

NEPAD. accessed August 26, 2010:
   http://www.nepad.org/documents/ (broken url)

OEDC. "Understanding the Digital Divide." OECD (Organisation for Economic Co-operation and Development), 2001.

Stally A., Ngwerume P. and Kimemiah P. "Readership Survey: Exchange on HIV/AIDS, Sexuality and Gender" 2009.

Wilson, T. "Electronic publishing and the future of the book: A paper delivered at the International Conference on Book Science to commemorate the 450th anniversary of the first Lithuanian book." Vilnius University, Lithuania, 24-28 September, 1997.

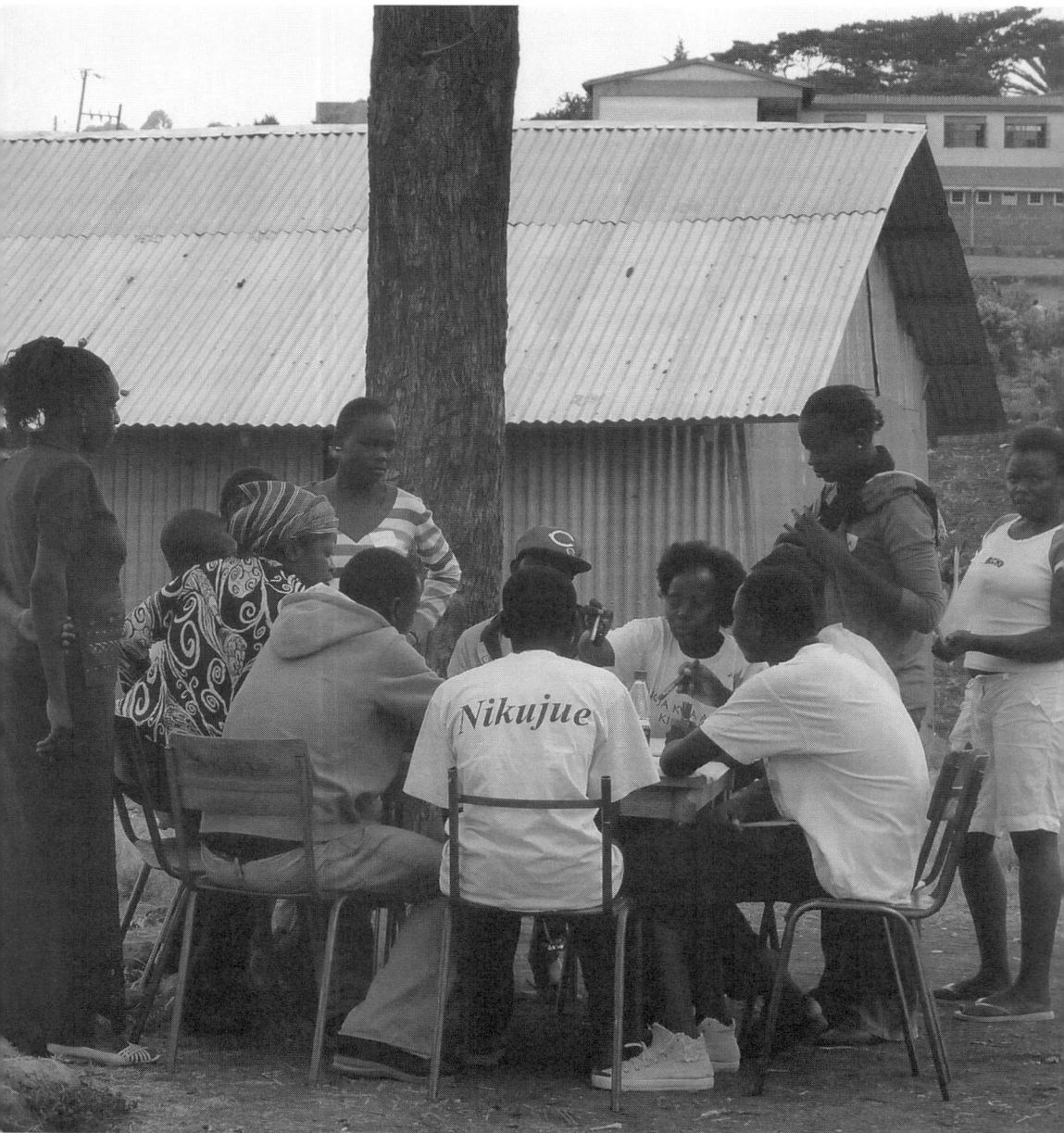

Sexual and reproductive desires and practices of Kenyan young positives: Opportunities for skills building through social media

Anke van der Kwaak, Francis Obare and Hermen Ormel

In this chapter the opportunities for skills building among HIV-positive adolescent boys and girls in Kenya through the use of social media to address their sexual and reproductive health (SRH) information and service needs will be discussed.[1] It is based on: (1) the findings of a diagnostic study conducted among adolescent boys and girls living with HIV in Kenya that assessed the SRH information and service needs of the adolescents with the aim of identifying and developing interventions that integrate these needs into the existing HIV and AIDS programmes (Obare and Van der Kwaak et al., 2010); (2) a workshop on Bridging and Bonding held on October 16-17 2010, in Kibera, Nairobi with 50 young people who took part in the diagnostic study; and (3) the work of the Netherlands-based Royal Tropical Institute (KIT) on mobile health (*mhealth*).[2]

The study among HIV-positive adolescents was implemented in Nairobi and Nyanza provinces in 2009 by Plan International-Kenya and KIT through funding from Plan International-Netherlands, KIT, and the Dutch Ministry of Foreign Affairs. KIT's work on *mhealth*, on the other hand, involves: (1) MobiScopy, a device that facilitates the use of a mobile phone camera to take and send microscopic images to an e-platform for remote diagnosis by a more experienced health worker; (2) a study into the feasibility of improving maternal health by enabling client-provider contact in emergencies, provider-client health promotion, and provider-provider communication to improve quality of care; and (3) the use of mobile phones to produce short project-related documentaries, and as an awareness and skills development tool for young people.

This chapter begins by presenting a summary of the relevant findings from the Kenyan study and their implications for programmatic actions as a way of identifying opportunities for the use of social media. It then highlights some of the existing challenges regarding SRH communication with young people, building self-esteem and life skills. Next, it outlines some of the examples of the use of social media and mobile phones to address public health issues and developments around the globe. It concludes by providing a brief description of the skills building and communication workshop for HIV-positive adolescents in Kenya using mobile phone technology.

---

[1] Social media is the use of internet- or mobile-based tools for social interaction, which is, sharing and discussing knowledge and information.
[2] Mobile health (mhealth) is the use of mobile communication and multimedia technology for public health and well-being.

Summary of study findings and implications

The diagnostic study involved a survey of 606 HIV-positive young people aged 15-19 years who were aware of their sero-status, and had a reflective ability to talk about their inner lives as well as four focus group discussions – comprising eight participants each – with a subset of the adolescents aged 18-19 years (Obare and Van der Kwaak et al., 2010). Study participants were identified and recruited through HIV and AIDS treatment, care and support centres with the help of counsellors, community health workers and social health workers. Female respondents comprised the majority (78%) of the study participants. This could partly be attributed to their greater vulnerability given that in Kenya, as elsewhere in sub-Saharan Africa, women are disproportionately affected by HIV and AIDS compared to men. It could also be due to better health-seeking behaviour among women than men. The study further found that most of the HIV-positive adolescents are vulnerable on account of several factors including their young age coupled with the fact that they are living with a chronic illness, many have lost one or both parents and the majority, especially the girls, are out of school. Moreover, only 50% belonged to any psychosocial support group (43% of the boys and 52% of the girls) (Obare and Van der Kwaak et al., 2010).

With respect to sexual and reproductive desires and practices, the findings show that most of the adolescents have already been in a sexual relationship (78% of the boys and 89% of the girls) while many of those who have never been in a sexual relationship intend to be involved in one in the future (97% of the boys and 84% of the girls). In addition, 84% of the respondents have already had sex (73% of the boys and 88% of the girls). Moreover, 76% of the adolescents intend to have children in future (90% of the boys and 73% of the girls) (Obare and Van der Kwaak et al., 2010). In summary, adolescents – whether HIV-positive or HIV-negative – desire to fall in love, have sex and plan for children.

However, most HIV and AIDS programmes dealing with HIV-positive adolescent clients focus on managing illness. Service providers do not seem to be interested, motivated or prepared to find out whether these clients are dating and are sexually active in order to provide appropriate SRH information and services (Obare and Van der Kwaak et al., 2010). Whereas there are efforts to integrate reproductive health and HIV services, these tend to focus on adults. Moreover, although some HIV and AIDS treatment, care and support programmes have incorporated child counselling into their packages, this falls short of mentioning sexuality, social empowerment and rights issues. Thus, HIV-positive adolescents are not empowered with the necessary information to enable them to balance rights and responsibilities, make informed decisions about relationships and sex, and achieve a higher quality of life in general.

Based on the findings of the study, some of the recommendations for programmatic actions included the need to (Obare and Van der Kwaak et al., 2010):
- update the existing counselling and support packages to include SRH information and services in order to equip service providers/counsellors with a tool to systematically assess the SRH needs of HIV-positive adolescents, and to address such needs in time or make appropriate referral;
- encourage and strengthen support groups for HIV-positive adolescents as these are a source of peer and psychosocial support, life skills training, and potential avenues for channelling SRH information;

- strengthen life skills training for HIV-positive adolescents to enable them to make informed choices, and to balance responsibility with sexual and reproductive desires and rights.

The above findings and implications suggest that involvement of HIV-positive young people in social programmes that address their aspirations and rights in the context of chronic illness and vulnerability are needed.

Challenges with sexual and reproductive health communication

As already noted, most HIV and AIDS programmes focus on managing illness and fail to appreciate the fact that HIV-positive young people have different aspirations in life including being successful in their careers, marrying, and having children. This could be partly due to social, cultural and religious norms in most parts of sub-Saharan Africa that do not sanction adolescent sexuality and childbearing, and guide the discussion of adolescent SRH issues (Marston and King, 2006; Mturi and Moerane, 2001). It could also be due to lack of appropriate training on the part of the service providers to offer SRH information and counselling to HIV-positive adolescents ((Birungi, Obare and Mugisha et al., 2009; Birungi, Mugisha and Nyombi et al., 2008). This suggests the need for innovative strategies for addressing SRH issues, empowerment, self-esteem, desires and professional aspirations of HIV-positive adolescents within programmes.

The other challenge stems from the multiple layered identities of young people in general, which makes dealing with adolescent SRH issues a complex task. For instance, young people's behaviour has been found to be context-specific, voicing certain normative attitudes in school while espousing alternative attitudes and behaviours in other contexts (Mitchell, Halpern and Kamathi, 2006; Nzioka 2001). This 'repertoire of faces' seems a necessary coping strategy for young people and might imply that HIV-positive adolescents included in the Kenyan study show different attitudes and behaviours depending on the context, but are also treated differently in different contexts. The enacted and perceived stigma that HIV-positive young people face may interlock with their identities of being a young girl or boy, going to school, being an orphan, and involuntary disclosure of HIV status. This complex, often conflicting and confusing reality in which young people live and in which they follow their aspirations underscores the need for supporting them with life-skills, communication skills, as well as coping strategies that go beyond disclosure or communicating about their illness.

Social media and mobile phones for public health and development

Accessible web-based technologies are used for creation and exchange of user-generated content. Common examples are the popular social networking sites like *Facebook* and *MySpace* but also include *YouTube, Flickr, Twitter, Wikipedia*, blogs and chat sites. Social media are increasingly being used for public health and social development purposes by embedding them in specific, interactive websites and web-based networks. However, computer-based web access is still limited for most people in many developing countries, especially those outside urban areas, due to limited bandwidth and prohibitive costs. In contrast, mobile phone access and coverage are rapidly expanding.

Standard mobile phones have at least voice, voicemail and short message service (sms) or text options, and often a camera for photos/video and multimedia messaging service (mms) while smart phones have e-mail and web access. In recent years, mobile communication and

multimedia technology are increasingly being used for *mhealth* in order to improve public health and well-being. Expectations for the potential impact of *mhealth* are high in terms of increasing access to information and services, improving quality, and lowering cost of services. Mobile phones have also rapidly become a popular tool in the broader field of development-related communication and social networking. Some examples of mobile phone and social media use in HIV and AIDS programmes include:
- The *Sex::Tech 2010*, a US-based sexuality conference focused on social media and mobile technology using *Twitter*, *Flickr*, *Facebook*, *YouTube* and blogs. According to *Sex::Tech* (ISIS, 2010), "The Internet and mobile technologies have strengthened youth networks, provided new avenues for expression, and increased youth access to tools and information designed to improve their sexual health. *Sex::Tech* explores available tools and methods for reaching youth with culturally-appropriate STD/HIV prevention and sex education interventions."
- The *LoveLife-Youth* project/network in South Africa reports connecting more than 6,000 peer educators to 5,100 schools, 150 community-based organisations (CBOs) and 500 clinics with 500,000 youth not only on a face-to-face basis but also through chat rooms, quizzes, and the cell phone-based social network, *MYMsta*, which has 45,000 registered users.
- The Dutch non-governmental organisation, *Text to Change*, sent interactive HIV awareness quizzes to 15,000 mobile subscribers in Uganda. This led to a 40% increase in clients who came in for testing – from 1,000 to 1,400 – during a six-week period (TTC, 2008).
- In South Africa, *Cell-life* uses mobile phones for behaviour change communication and HIV treatment adherence support. As De Tolly and Alexander (2009) note, "The opportunities in South Africa for using mobile technologies to support initiatives in the HIV and AIDS sector are enormous. A huge number of people have cell phone access, and there are a range of innovative ways in which cell phones can be used to support treatment, disseminate information, provide anonymous counselling, gather data, and link patients to services."

Mechael and colleagues (2010: 69) have reviewed present approaches in *mhealth*. They conclude that "the mobile technologies when applied to addressing health issues… are beginning to gain traction and show positive, albeit mixed results," and that for the "programmes to succeed, an enabling well-informed policy and business environment that engages all relevant public and private health and IT stakeholders to drive scale and sustainability is needed."

Skills building and communication workshop in Kenya
A post-research workshop took place in Kibera, Nairobi as a follow-up programme aimed at engaging young people living with HIV face-to-face as well as through virtual communication as a channel for addressing their SRH information and service needs[3]. Its objectives were to:
- Enhance the understanding and skills of the participants to use mobile technology and social media, in order to increase self-esteem and life skills and strengthen 'bonding' activities (among themselves and with other young positives) and 'bridging' efforts (with other groups such as parents, other adolescents, and service providers) for positive living, improved quality of life, and exercising of rights;

---

[3] This activity was funded by Plan Netherlands and the Dutch Royal Tropical Institute.

- Improve participants' ability to discuss their desires and dreams in terms of social relations; bonding and bridging; positive living and quality of life; exercising rights; information use; and social responsibilities;
- Provide participants with an opportunity to discuss options, benefits and personal interest regarding the use of mobile phones and social media related to their aspirations, identities, and dreams as well as to develop and implement simple ideas for use of mobile phones and possibly other media.

The workshop also aimed at using new approaches to facilitate life skills training for HIV-positive young people in Kenya and to use mobile technology and social media as exciting ways of attracting and engaging them in topics such as HIV prevention and care, as well as rights-based development of self-esteem. It involved mind mapping exercises, representations on power and self-esteem, the presentation of short state-of-the-art social media approaches and a description of the intentions to use these approaches in the work with young people. Managed by a local NGO involved in work with youth and social media (Nairobits), a Facebook page was established during the workshop to enable communication, sharing and community building among the 50 young participants as well as representatives of the Foundation of People living with HIV and AIDS in Kenya (FOPHAK), AMREF and mobilisers of treatment centres. Workshop outputs (mind maps, poster representations on self-esteem) as well as selected photos were immediately uploaded on the Facebook page.

Mobile technology was used as a tool for motivation and communication, later to be integrated with social media. On several occasions during and after the workshops bulk text messages (sms) with motivational contents and questions were sent out to all participants, generating reasonable (>50%) response levels. A subsequent workshop will be held early 2011. The work will be undertaken with the organisations mentioned above, the Kenyan government, and service providers working with HIV-positive adolescents. Liverpool VCT and other organisations are eager to participate. A series of workshops and other initiatives are envisaged to respond to these young people's rights and needs. The workshop showed that there is an urgent need for knowledge and information about sexuality and HIV-related issues among the young people; and that mobile technology, the Internet and social media have a highly motivational quality for young people and are potentially effective assets for channelling information and addressing self-reflection, monitoring and evaluation, and community-building for mutual support; and identifying and engaging other key stakeholders in the process.

Forging ahead
This chapter highlights some of the findings and recommendations of a diagnostic study and related life-skills workshop that assessed the SRH information and service needs of young people living with HIV in Kenya with a view to identifying opportunities for the use of social media to address some of these needs. The findings of the diagnostic study show that the SRH needs of HIV-positive young people require social programmes that address their aspirations and rights in the context of chronic illness and vulnerability. Coupled with the challenges of dealing with adolescent SRH issues in general, there is a need for innovative strategies – such as the use of social media – to address issues of SRH, empowerment, self-esteem, desires and professional aspirations of HIV-positive adolescents within HIV and AIDS programmes.

Acknowledgements

The authors would like to acknowledge the contributions of Bwibo Adieri, David Owuor, Stephen Okoth, Samuel Musyoki, Emily Muga, and Harriet Birungi to the diagnostic study among HIV-positive adolescents in Kenya. The study also benefited from technical input from Jet Bastiani and Korrie de Koning, and logistical support from the Provincial Medical Officer- Nyanza, the Provincial Children's Officer- Nairobi, the District Children's Officers- Nairobi, and the Medical Officer of Health- City Council of Nairobi. Eliezer Wangulu provided valuable comments on an earlier version of this chapter.

Furthermore, the authors thank Maureen Khaniri and Tobias Ouma for their important role in organising and co-facilitating the workshop.

References

Birungi H., F. Obare and J.F. Mugisha et al. "Preventive service needs of young people perinatally infected with HIV in Uganda." In: *AIDS Care* 21(2009)6: p. 725-731.

Birungi H., J.F. Mugisha and J. Nyombi et al. "Sexual and reproductive health needs of adolescents perinatally infected with HIV in Uganda." In: *FRONTIERS Final Report*. Washington, DC: Population Council, 2008.

ISIS. Sex::Tech Conference 2011 website. accessed 31 August 2010: http://www.sextech.org/

Marston C. and E. King. "Factors that shape young people's sexual behaviour: A systematic review." In: *Lancet,* 368(2006)9547: p. 1581-1586.

Mechael P., H. Batavia and N. Kaonga, et al. "Barriers and Gaps Affecting mHealth in Low and Middle Income Countries: Policy White Paper." New York: Centre for Global Health and Economic Development Earth Institute, Columbia University, 2010.

Mitchell E., M.H.C.T. Halpern and E.M. Kamathi. "Social scripts and stark realities: Kenyan adolescents' abortion discourse." In: *Culture, Health & Sexuality*, 8(2006)6: p. 515-528.

Mturi A.J. and W. Moerane. "Premarital childbearing among adolescents in Lesotho." In: *Journal of Southern African Studies,* 27(2001)2: p. 259-275.

Nzioka C. "Perspectives of adolescent boys on the risks of unwanted pregnancy and sexually transmitted infections: Kenya." In: *Reproductive Health Matters,* 9(2001)17: p. 108-117.

Obare F., and A. van der Kwaak, et al. "HIV-positive adolescents in Kenya: Access to sexual and reproductive health services." Amsterdam: KIT Publishers, 2010.

Tolly K. de, and H. Alexander. "Innovative use of cellphone technology for HIV and AIDS behaviour change communications: Three Pilot Projects." Cellphones4HIV, March, 2009. accessed 31 August 2010: http://mobileactive.org/research/innovative-use-cell-phone-technology-hiv-aids-behaviour-change-communications-3-pilot-proje

TTC (Text to Change). "Identifying the Building Blocks for Sustainable and Scalable mHealth Programs: Uganda." TTC, 2008. accessed 31 August 2010: http://www.texttochange.com/mHealth_for_Development_TTC.pdf

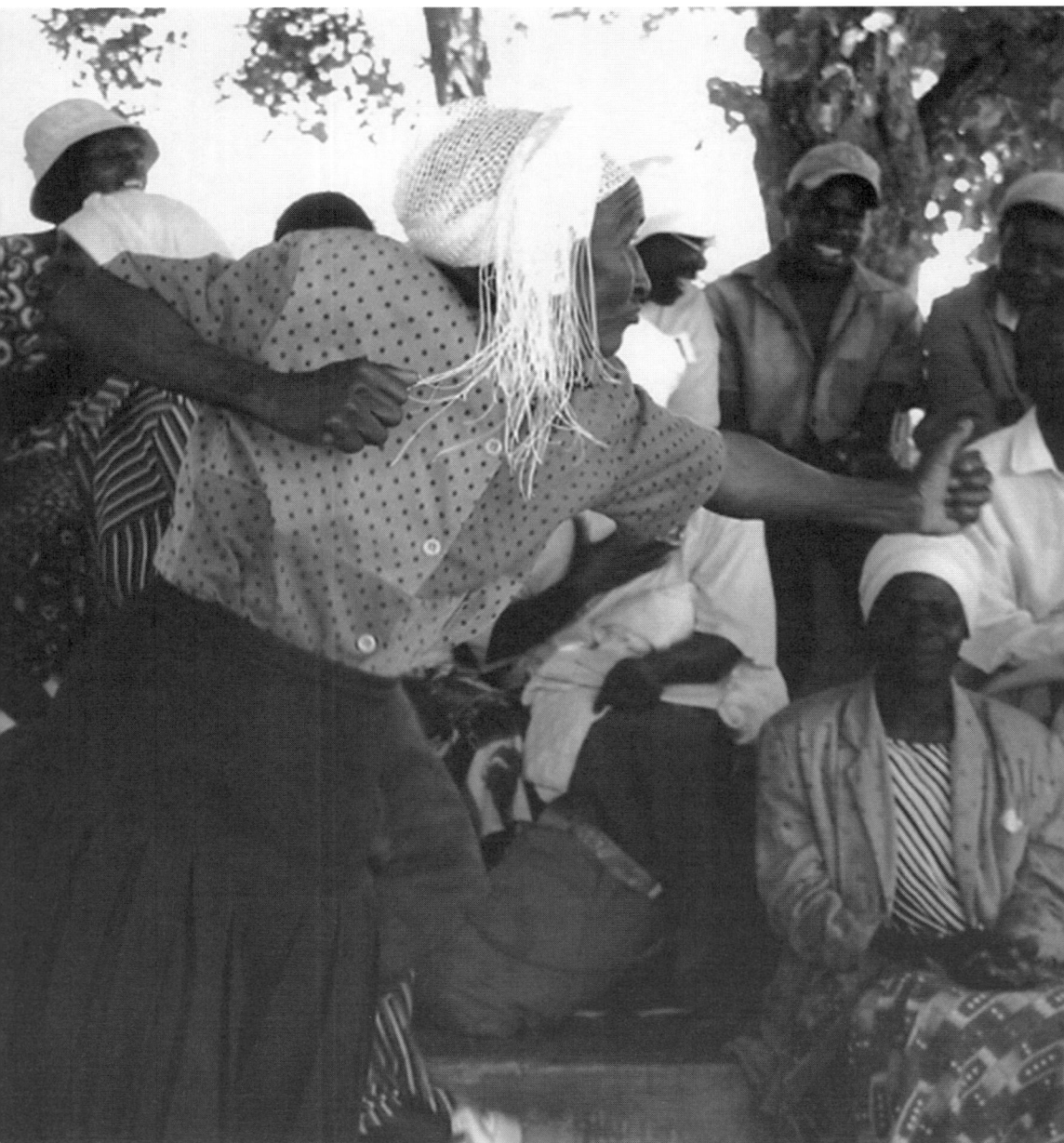

Monitoring and Evaluation: Measuring for change

Jan Reynders

This chapter examines socio-cultural dynamics of monitoring and evaluation (M&E) of change processes that address the linkages of gender-based violence >< education >< culture >< HIV prevention. We shall review participatory M&E processes that can assist organisations active in these fields to measure and assess their work and thus to organise their internal learning, feedback and reporting systems and simultaneously to be accountable to their funding partners for the financial contributions received.

While M&E can be considered an indispensable tool for change towards equity and justice, it is also a tremendous challenge. As long-time independent gender and development consultant and as former staff member of a northern funding agency, often engaged in M&E processes in both functions, I have come across not only considerable confusion and unnecessary anxieties about assessments, but also encouraging examples of how evaluation can be an empowering experience and how 'measuring can be a tool for change'. In this chapter I shall share what I have learned over time regarding the 'what' and the 'how' of the 'culture of M&E' and argue for a participatory approach to measuring change, fully-owned by the people and institutions involved. I also discuss some of the issues and concerns with respect to M&E and the position and roles of donors in funding relations that were raised in the Cross-cultural Learning Conference held in Johannesburg in South Africa in April 2010 on the linkages between culture, gender-based violence, education and HIV prevention.[1]

Evaluations are often feared: time to review the ownership and skills

For many civil society organisations (CSOs) that receive financial support from funding agencies in the global north, the thought of an external evaluation easily puts chills down the spine. Why is that so? Why are external evaluations not seen as part of internal learning and feedback processes that NGOs need themselves to assess whether and how they do - or do not - make a difference, how they contribute to the change they want to promote? And why does internal monitoring and evaluation often only get low priority in the time allocated for staff members? Both funding agencies and NGOs receiving their funding have their own approaches and experiences with respect to external evaluations. Some of their interests are shared, related to the common objectives of their partnership, some are different, related to the unequal positions they hold in the power relation - 'funders have the money, the recipients want it' - as well as the structures and requirements for public accountability.

The fear that many NGOs have with respect to external evaluations or M&E in general can thus relate to the ownership of the evaluation process, based on their marginal power

---

[1] In this chapter I shall refer to different types of evaluations and monitoring processes as tools for assessment: external evaluations; externally facilitated internal evaluations; internal evaluation and similarly organised forms of monitoring processes. It goes beyond the scope of this chapter to go into details about these different forms of organising M&E.

position vis-à-vis the funding agency, but it can also be attributed to their lack of capacity, not knowing how to measure or show what – however intangible – contributions to change they were able to make. Many donor agencies fail to recognise the enormous diversity among their receiving partners in the levels of understanding about M&E and the skills required to organise meaningful M&E.

Fear about evaluations often relates to the experiences that organisations or individuals have had with earlier evaluations. Many evaluations - sadly enough - have been and are even today undertaken as inspections rather than as participatory assessments, in which the evaluated organisation has as many positive stakes as the funding partner with whom the evaluation is agreed. Certainly, if there is a programme to construct a bridge, drill a hundred boreholes for drinking water or construct 200 school buildings, there is the element of inspection: have the constructions all been completed according to specifications, within the specified budgets and time and according to agreed processes of (participatory) planning? But when a CSO has a programme of delivering HIV-awareness training to particular community groups, or implements a date-rape prevention programme addressing boys and girls through local schools, or addresses gender-based violence (GBV) e.g. through a women's empowerment programme, inspections cannot provide the needed feedback for accountability, nor can they cover the wealth of experiences and lessons to be learned and taken forward. Traditional notions of power, hierarchy and leadership and even ideological baggage from the past may also lead to fear of evaluations. In many countries formerly under the influence of the then Soviet Union for example, the word evaluation is simply equated with inspection.

If indeed implementation of programmes has always merely been inspected, rather than assessed for its progress, output and outcome and if that has directly related to the availability of further funding and hence salaries to employ staff, understandably there is fear: "what if we have not reached the expected numbers, output or quality?", "What if we have not lived up to the expectations of the funders in this HIV prevention programme?" Of course there are weaknesses in every programme and every organisation, but is it wise to show that? How much will be noticed, how much can better be hidden, if it is likely to have direct consequences for future funding and hence staff positions? Many NGOs receiving donor funding have experienced themselves, or know from others, how some donors have indeed used weaknesses in their outcome as justification to terminate funding. Many organisations therefore tend to downplay or even hide the weaknesses, whether during evaluations, programme visits or progress reporting, particularly when activities are not easily 'tangible' like empowerment, HIV awareness or changed attitudes and behaviour. Yet everyone knows that no organisation or programme is perfect.

The fear of external evaluations, whether conducted with local evaluators or those from outside the region, is often based on many unknown factors related to expectations. What norms and indicators of success are used in the assessment? Whose norms are they? What baseline was there against which assessment takes place? Is an increase of GBV or HIV prevalence an indication of the failure of a programme? What understanding of the local setting does the evaluation team have, and for that matter the NGO implementing the programme as well, if sensitive cultural issues are at play: sex and patriarchal power, boys and girls, women and men, abuse and submission. This is particularly important in relation to the role of and respect for traditional leadership, religious practices, gender relations, ethnic hierarchies and interpretations of sexual and reproductive rights or sexual and other diversity issues. Are patriarchal traditions accepted as the norm or are they being questioned? What – if anything – has been agreed at the start of the programme that would be addressed or changed and hence measured e.g. in terms of unequal gender power relations, male dominance, attitudes towards consensual sex, HIV infection prevention behaviour? Who was involved in taking those decisions?

Many NGOs have to deal with changing staff and changing views, policies and priorities of their (northern) funding partners and hence easily feel that the expectations are changing over time without being adequately discussed or negotiated. Other or newly appointed programme officers of the funding agencies often also bring their personal views, which is often rather different from the earlier programme officer. Having to deal with three or four donor agency programme officers in the span of just a few years is not exceptional! Many organisations receiving external funding do not feel strong enough to question such changed organisational or personal expectations and views and rather quietly comply with new priorities, rules, norms or reporting systems, imposed by the different funders. Many such NGOs will even claim expertise and compliance with new policies and approaches of funders - like the focus on gender justice or HIV prevention - in order to secure continued funding[2]. Cynically, NGOs refer at times to the "fashion-of-the-year" of the northern funders[3]: certainly not a good basis for an honest partnership between funders and fund recipients. I have noted that only CSOs that feel strong enough on the basis of their own work experience, conviction and M&E expertise and that have multiple funding sources, are able (and have the courage) to follow their own line of planning, programming and progress reporting, rather than giving in to donor pressure for their survival. They certainly discuss new views and preferences of funders but only incorporate new ideas where considered appropriate.

The importance of M&E: measuring (for) change
Why evaluate anyway? Measuring to produce change or measuring the changes produced? Or both? Among the more activist style NGOs, there is a tendency to underestimate the importance of monitoring and evaluating, whether internal or facilitated from outside. Many NGOs argue that they are busy campaigning, motivating and supporting community groups against sexual abuse and equal rights of women or training specific categories like youngsters, poor women or sex workers towards their awareness and empowerment to prevent HIV infections or providing services to them to the best of their ability. They do all of this with limited means, a small staff and many volunteers: why spend time on recording activities and measuring outputs or outcome? For many organisations record keeping is done only to satisfy the funding agencies. Programme log frames prepared as condition for funding are often not seen as supportive monitoring tools, but as a nuisance imposed by funders. Many NGOs argue that the situation and circumstances they work in are unique and hence no evaluation norm or standard is applicable: they should simply be allowed to work hard.

---

[2] There was a strong feeling at the conference that money should follow programmes and not programmes to follow funds. Meaning NGOs or implementers should not venture into areas they do not have expertise in just because they want the money. On the other hand, donors should be sensitive to the local needs and provide funds without being so stringent on what they should fund.

[3] For example anyone active in the broad field of (the right to) health care has witnessed the major shift in funding a number of years ago from malaria and tuberculosis prevention to HIV and AIDS prevention. As if malaria and tuberculosis had ceased to be the primary cause of death among the poor in many regions of the world.

While the notion of the specific and difficult, perhaps even unique circumstances is indeed important, it cannot be a reason for an organisation not to engage in relevant M&E process. The emotion of 'doing good' does not automatically imply 'doing it well' and this emotion can never suffice for an organisation to continue without adequate reflection on how to 'do it well' step-by-step.

One organisation that had worked in different parts of Ethiopia for a long time had to conclude about its own limited learning capacity or willingness: 'yes, we have learned our lessons well: we repeat the same mistakes over and over again'.

Any organisation using public funds, whether raised locally or from international funders needs to account for the funds' usage. That is a formal requirement[4]. But at least equally important to remain relevant in their field: every organisation also needs to reflect on its actions, strategies, skills and output for its own learning. What was effective and relevant at the start of the organisation, in terms of strategy, activities, choice of clientele or staff skills, may not be sufficient or even justified any longer/more under changed circumstances. Government policies and services may have changed for better or worse, or the governance systems, health care services, education or the security situation may be different now and hence calling for a different response from the NGO. In weakened states impunity may have increased, affecting the most vulnerable members of the community. Economic circumstances have changed, sometimes there may be increased employment, but in many places as a result of the economic crisis there is a lack of employment opportunities both nearby and in faraway places[4]. All this impacts on the communities' and individuals' behaviour at home and in the migrant labour settings. The prevalence of GBV and rape may have increased as it indeed has in many places, often directly related to job insecurity for men, reversed migration, increased informal labour particularly employing women, who then become the main income earner, subsequently often with a crisis in masculinity notions of their partners, easily followed by substance abuse and violence. In turn, increased GBV easily leads to an increase in the prevalence of HIV infections. With increasing numbers of people migrating to urban areas the roles of traditional leadership in handling violence, sexual abuse and rape in communities has diminished. This results in changes in the need for and nature of campaigns, services and training, as well as in the scope to positively engage traditional leaders. Such shifts can only come to light if regular M&E takes place.

No society is static, and to continue programmes without regular reflection on their relevance, quality and effectiveness may easily lead to a waste of human and other resources, frustration among staff and diminishing public (and donor) support. It ultimately undermines the reason to exist as NGO. Uniqueness of situations therefore is no excuse to dismiss M&E.

> It is quite complex yet essential to monitor and evaluate the relevance, efficacy and effectiveness of an NGO as change agent in a setting which is changing anyway and in which change is thus both cause and effect of the problems related to GBV and unsafe sex. Hence I conclude: measuring of change is indispensable for change.

---

[4] Particularly migrant labour workers, working in faraway, often foreign countries, both seasonal and longer term e.g. in mines and construction sites, have been hit hard with unemployment and needed to go back home or stay put and live on minimal savings waiting for better times.

If an NGO is set up to bring about a particular change, to promote gender justice, to reduce HIV prevalence, or address the exclusion of people living with HIV and AIDS, there is a continuous need to measure its progress, effectiveness, outcome and the role that traditional cultural practices play in that, both positive and harmful, and make changes when required: NGOs need to measure for change.

Designing internal M&E systems: how to measure what works and what does not
Reluctance or even resistance within organisations to M&E processes needs to be analysed for its causes. Particularly when external circumstances have changed considerably, staff may feel that monitoring of output and outcome of activities may expose weaknesses of the programme and the staff's capacities and call for changes. Given the common tendency of many people and organisations to resist change, which requires moving out of existing comfort zones of known processes, systems and ways of working, M&E systems need to be carefully designed, planned and implemented, involving staff and – depending on the circumstances and activities – the clientele/communities. A safe space needs to be created to minimise resistance. From the highest level of the organisation importance must be placed on M&E processes to guarantee that staff will make adequate time available. Having an M&E system in place, even with a staff member recruited specifically for this job, but without adequate acknowledgement of its importance by the management and positive support from the staff, will not work: M&E needs to become part of job descriptions, staff routines and time use allocation. If activity feedback reporting, entering data in (electronic) reporting systems, including baseline data collection, internal review sessions, or case studies are organised as 'on top of' rather than as 'part of' regular task performance, its quality will suffer and staff will be less motivated to make it work. The M&E system must be 'owned' by the staff and by the organisation as something useful for their (own) development, better performance or job satisfaction. That will obviously require that staff members are enabled to contribute to the system design, trained in its usage and see the added value for themselves. Regrettably that does not always happen.

M&E that only feeds the management with the data required for satisfying the funders, or which is primarily used to 'check' on staff performance without feedback and learning opportunities, is rarely performed with honesty. M&E systems need to be non-threatening in nature to get the staff support required. That does not mean that weaknesses in activities' implementation, limited output and outcome or weak performance of teams or individual staff members cannot be reported and addressed, whether the result of inadequate staffing, skills, work attitudes or supervision. In an atmosphere of trust and mutual support, weaknesses can be addressed as challenges to be resolved. In an atmosphere of distrust they may lead to disempowerment and fear e.g. of job security, humiliation.

> M&E cannot be done in isolation from the clientele that the NGOs work with, the community groups or specific groups of vulnerable women, students, migrants, informal sector workers and their new or traditional leaders, patrons or guardians, whose 'blessing' or active support is generally required to be acceptable. This is true in general but particularly when the work is related to culturally-sensitive issues such as gender-based violence and HIV prevention or education dealing with sex and sexuality, gender justice and girls and women's rights.

The changes in knowledge, awareness, assertiveness, self-protection, attitudes and behaviour are ultimately what matters in HIV prevention and gender justice promotion and the clientele itself needs to be involved in the assessments of the change processes. Not as mere data providers or showcase examples – community groups or schoolgirls that often get visited by funders easily feel objects, rather than subjects of the change processes – but as core participants in the assessment. Without their weighted reflections an activity may be rated positive by the NGO, without the clientele seeing any changes they hoped for! Hence programme and subsequently M&E designs need to incorporate the hopes and expectations of the clientele as well. It is the task of the NGO to capture the issues and problems the clientele likes to see addressed and changed (stopping violence and rape, men taking responsibility for their behaviour, fatherhood responsibilities, etc) and translate these into campaigns, training and services with indicators of success that reflect the expectations as expressed by the clientele.

External evaluations: how can they be turned into empowering experiences?
Similar to the design of internal M&E systems, external evaluations, whether as an initiative of the NGO itself or at the request of funding partners, must be based on an agenda that is acceptable to all stakeholders. Even if the request has come from the (foreign) funding partner as part of the funding conditions, the fund-receiving partner must have clear stakes in the evaluation as well. Without an acceptable common agenda for both partners, honest data collection for a useful assessment of performance, output and outcome cannot be expected. This would reduce the evaluation to a mere inspection for upward accountability purposes.

> "Different positions of power are everywhere and need to be recognised for the way they influence plans, policies, practices, priority setting and evaluations. Yet the donor >< recipient NGO relation needs to be based on trust. But trust needs to be built and maintained. This requires time, open dialogue and honest M&E." (A participant in the M&E workshop during the Johannesburg conference).

The role of the funding partner needs to be assessed as well, particularly if the funding agency claims to be more than just a grant-maker. Hence assessing the partnership and roles of each partner must be included in the terms of reference (ToR) for the evaluation. Ideally an evaluation thus includes learning opportunities for both organisations e.g. in terms of any planned or unplanned networking, experience exchanges or knowledge and method sharing.

The development of the ToR for an external evaluation is an important part of the start-up process as it gives the space for the stakeholders to get each of their different agendas discussed and – to the extent agreed – included in the final ToR. But we need to be realistic as well. Given the workload, the task divisions and the skills in many NGOs, it is unlikely that many staff members are involved in the development of, or in discussing a draft ToR for an external evaluation. More often than not the draft ToR is prepared by the donor agency single-handedly. Some donor agencies are also not very keen to allow time and space for negotiating the ToR content or the process, is initiated at such a late hour that a participatory process is not feasible. Given the unequal power relation between funders and fund recipient organisations, the receivers may simply accept a ToR as drafted by the donor, even if they are not happy about it. This can be rather frustrating particularly for funding agencies' staff members who are keen to engage in open dialogues.

> **Fear turning into an empowering process**
> Late 2009 an NGO in South Africa was very unhappy with the tone, assumptions and prior negative 'conclusions' in the draft ToR for an external evaluation they had received from the donor. But the board of the NGO instructed the director to accept the ToR as it came, for fear of repercussions by the donor if they disagreed with the formulations. The ToR remained in draft status. Before starting the actual evaluation process the NGO staff team and evaluator reviewed the formulations, removed assumptions and jointly reformulated the same issues into research questions that were relevant for the NGO's fact finding and learning process.

For an evaluation to be an empowering experience, the composition of the evaluation team is of vital importance. A quite common approach in a two-member team in external evaluations is to have one member proposed by the donor agency and one by the recipient. While it is positive to draw on the diverse networks of contacts of either partner, it only works well if the proposed evaluators are and can function truly independent of the donor and recipient respectively, rather than defend or represent the interests of either organisation. The issues to be covered need to come from an accepted ToR, not from hidden agendas.

In this field of sensitive issues of GBV, rape and other abuse, sexuality attitudes, HIV, male dominance, gender relations, diversity issues, cultural and religious traditions, it is of great importance to make sure the evaluation team brings in adequate experience, skills and sensitivity to deal with these issues. I have seen colleagues put forward for evaluation teams who never dealt with any issues of violence or rape, and for whom discussing issues around sex and particularly homosexuality was very uncomfortable or even taboo. Given that gender injustice, abuse, or HIV prevention by its very nature mostly deals with women and men, it is advisable in most situations to have a sex-mixed team.

It is certainly possible to make an evaluation assignment participatory and self-reflective and thus an empowering experience for all involved. In the appendix to this chapter I briefly describe the basic principles and elements of the process that I usually follow when an external evaluation is initiated by the funding agency as part of the existing funding contract. These apply particularly in the field of HIV prevention/GBV where the progress that can be made is slow and of which the evidence is difficult to establish.
Such a process includes not only organising workshops with the relevant staff and board of the NGO to initiate and conclude the evaluation process, it also includes reviewing the scope and limits of the donor role. I prefer to de-link the evaluation process from the funding decision moments, but this is often difficult to accomplish as most external evaluations are planned near the termination of a funding phase and are thus easily seen as an 'exam' that determines the future (levels of) funding[5].

---

[5] I have had to refuse evaluation assignments where the funding agency already had decided that they would stop funding because, based on their own short visits, they were not satisfied with the NGO's performance, but they wanted the evaluator to 'conclude' the same and give that message to the NGO.

Monitoring and measuring the immeasurable

Much of what has been discussed so far in terms of culturally-sensitive participatory evaluation processes is applicable and useful in many other fields of development as well. What makes M&E different in the context of the linkages between culture, GBV, education and HIV prevention is the nature of the changes that are hoped for and worked on: changes in human behaviour, expressions of sexuality and gender justice: men turning their masculinity into positive and responsible behaviour, taking full responsibility for their behaviour in relating to their partners and themselves. It also means men taking responsibility in their fatherhood roles, ending abuse in relations, stopping rape and preventing the spread of HIV. It also includes women empowering themselves to take charge of their own lives, preventing vulnerability to abuse and rape. It also refers to children, girls and boys, safely and happily living their youth life, getting educated and groomed to become responsible adult women and men living respectful, happy and gender-just lives. NGOs often intend to promote all this through education, training, awareness campaigns and support services, using the power of positive cultural traditions and new (women) leadership, or role models.

Most of these changes are rather intangible and seemingly immeasurable. So what do we measure in order to know whether progress is made? There is no one handbook for the 'right' and adequate way of doing these things. Moreover how do we discern the change brought about by the NGO amidst the overall changes taking place? Circumstances are always specific and also change over time: attitudes of people change, governments change their policies, power relations change, job options too. As indicated before, also the strength of some cultural traditions (which may include strong notions of leadership, conflict resolution practices, rites of passage to adulthood with training about the values and responsibilities that come with this) as well as social control mechanisms to protect the respect for certain values have changed and weakened with increased migration, urbanisation and the globalisation of cultures.

There have been and still are many harmful cultural practices as well, particularly endangering the health, well-being and rights of girls and women, like girl-child marriages, sometimes even promoted by religious leaders of particular sects. There is also the strong widespread myth in a number of countries that grew out of ignorance about the origins of HIV and AIDS, that having sex with a virgin will cure AIDS and hence many young girls get raped and infected. Some of the myths, beliefs and practices are very strong and were based on or have become new elements of the overall male dominance found in most societies.

What does all this mean for M&E in the field of HIV prevention and gender justice? First of all that it is a difficult task in the context of a time-bound project of a few years to indicate, let alone prove or confirm, what the contribution has been by an NGO, through its campaigns, training, counselling to reduce HIV infection, stop GBV or enhance gender justice and women's rights. Much of the work done does not have immediate effects but will – if indeed useful/successful – show only after some time. If GBV is not reduced during the project period, if rape has not stopped, or if the incidence of HIV infection has not been reduced, can the project be considered a failure?

Causal linkages between education, campaigns and other activities in relation to GBV/gender justice and HIV prevention - whether focussing on sexual abuse, domestic violence or HIV infection and subsequent stigmatisation/victimisation - in society and the actual reduction of infections/or absence of abuse of women and girls cannot be easily established. The influence of awareness-raising, training, empowerment efforts, attitude change, or for that matter new criminal laws and government policies, is slow and many other forces are at play influencing behaviour leading to/continuing or condoning violence, abuse, rape, etc. Hence evaluations and monitoring processes will need to look at the quality of the strategies and the added value of activities undertaken that may contribute to attitude change, awareness and actual prevention of HIV infections/GBV.

> Rather than looking for a one-to-one cause and effect chain, we need to assess the plausibility -rather than causality- of contributions to the envisaged change.

It does mean that NGOs cannot claim great success in a campaign, simply by virtue of the fact that lots of people have shown up for a rally, which got covered by the media; if hundreds of leaflets have been distributed or when many people have attended awareness training programmes. Attendance figures for meetings or training sessions are important but do not suffice. Claims of success and the roles played by the NGO and its programme need to be substantiated. Hence evaluations need to assess what can be established as the 'most significant change' (MSC) contributed through the work undertaken.

In many ways M&E of the social change that is required to redress HIV infections related to GBV, gender injustices, harmful traditional/cultural practices or non-acceptance of diverse sexual preference, meets with the same problems that (global) social change networks face: how to prove that your work has made a dent. Big programmes to sink bore-holes, build primary schools or provide vaccinations are often organised along traditional almost 'military' ways of planning, implementing and evaluating: carefully co-ordinated, target-oriented interventions ('target groups'), managed via a centrally-controlled, maximum efficient, chain of command and authority. This 'military model' of thinking has heavily pervaded the ways of organising, planning and evaluating development activities and even the language commonly used by NGOs and funders to describe its processes. But social change cannot be produced this way. Similar to international social networks (like women's rights networks), NGOs working in the field of HIV prevention related to GBV, education, cultural traditions, need to address development and change differently. Social change activities are not intended to control or direct the actions of others, but rather to facilitate the understanding of power and its abuse and the awareness and empowerment of women and men to develop and implement their own strategies to change their behaviour, deal with their responsibilities as men and women, fathers and mothers, boys and girls (Imam, Matsvai and Reynders, 1998).

Hence indicators for monitoring progress and for evaluating output and outcome must be developed to show the added value of the NGO towards the desired social change, the plausibility of its contribution made towards such change, a/o based on the assessment of the strategy of audience selection, quality of the publications, content of the training, in-build testing of changed attitudes, follow-up to training and government policy and services' changes to the extent that was intended and lobbied for by the NGO or happened as side-effect. Indicators of present (baseline) and changed attitudes and behaviour have to be established, particularly where concrete changes are strived after. This relates to work in the communities (women and men), with cultural leaders at different levels (e.g. no longer sanctioning girl-child marriage, changes in rites of passage to adulthood), with policy makers (appointment of female and male police officers trained in abuse issues to deal with women and men respectively) or with other CSOs, with government service agencies or the media (on coverage of cases).

> An awareness programme in secondary schools near Johannesburg in South Africa intended to stop or at least reduce the frequent 'date rape', (a boy taking a girl out, paying for her drinks and demanding/expecting sex in return) certainly made the learners think and raise the economic power difference: after school time the boys earn a wage in supermarkets, the girls work at home, caring for their siblings, without payment. The girls involuntarily gave in to sex as the social norm, until they started questioning that in the awareness programmes. Regular visits to the same schools could help in documenting whether the changed understanding leads to change in practice, hence providing evidence for monitoring and evaluation purposes.

In the case of activities undertaken with specific groups, e.g. university students, community groups in specific locations, court magistrates, concrete indicators can best be developed together with the specified audience: what is the situation at present, what would they like to see happen and what would they consider indications of success. This requires agreement on the baseline: the situation now, what needs to change and what is seen as change.

> Take the case of the campaign 'Consent is sexy' undertaken by an NGO and a professional and also activist awareness-campaigns design company with students from the University of Witwatersrand in South Africa. The situation: there is a lot of un-consented sex among students, (mostly) demanded by boys, based on male dominance, assumed 'rights' after dating, inability to say 'no' by girls and non-acceptance by male students of a female student's 'no'. A few months were taken for the preparation of the campaign with the students as they had to debate and agree on each campaign poster slogan and picture to be used on their campus. That in itself helped debate and led to acceptable, yet very strong poster texts that leave no doubts about the messages. E.g. *"Sex with consent is sexy, sex without consent is rape"*. The campaign brought about much debate and acknowledgement of un-consented sex among students. As one result a person/office of confidence was set up on campus to hear and deal with rape cases and other forms of sexual abuse. The NGO and design company were asked to cover other campuses as well and repeat the campaign in the following years. Without the long preparation and direct input by the students of what they expected to be addressed the campaign would not have been feasible. Lesson learned: in other campuses students will have to go through similar debate and slogan formulation exercises: simply spreading the slogans would not work, nor would it be acceptable. In terms of M&E purposes this means that the strategy of developing the campaign content and process needs to be recorded and assessed, as well as the student views on consent in sex prior to and some time after the campaign.

In order to be strategic and effective in their work, NGOs working in these difficult fields of HIV prevention through changing attitudes, sexual behaviour or gender power relations, need to be very concrete and develop short and longer-term objectives, strategies and activities directly relating to what they and the communities/clientele served expect as outputs. A baseline must be established with the clientele at the start of an activity as well as a monitoring process with indicators for the changes wanted and expected and considered relevant by the groups served. For effective NGO work in this difficult field more is needed than organising campaigns and awareness-raising trainings.

Conclusion

Measuring of change is indispensable for change: positive outcome cannot simply be assumed to happen when a dedicated NGO works hard. It is a must, particularly in the field of changing attitudes and behaviour and addressing patriarchal norms and negative notions of masculinity and male privileges that perpetuate violence against women, to continuously measure – M&E – the effectiveness of strategies chosen, audience selected, empowerment training or other support given.
Public funding money needs to be accounted for to the donors for its agreed and effective usage. For public accountability and acceptance NGOs need to be transparent about the funds they receive and how these are spent. Evaluations are thus a formal requirement when using public funds. But evaluations are of equal importance and an absolute necessity to the NGO itself to provide feedback internally on progress made and lessons to be learned in the processes of change.

Whether for accountability or internal learning purposes, and whether or not donor initiated, evaluations can be organised as empowering rather than fearsome experiences for all involved. For that to happen, the process of M&E and evaluations needs to be participatory, democratic and fully owned by the NGO. NGOs need to invest in their own capacity for M&E and self-evaluation. M&E will thus become part of the management approach and staff work routine, with adequate time allocation for data collection and processing, reporting, reflection and feedback sessions.
Measuring the 'immeasurable' desired and expected changes in attitudes and behaviour must be organised in participatory ways, involving the clientele or community groups to jointly establish baselines and indicators for the 'most significant changes'.
Only when M&E and evaluations are appreciated, at individual and institutional level, as supportive and indispensable, can these become effective tools for change.
Let us not assume to be effective: let us really measure for a change!

External evaluation as empowering experience

It is certainly possible to make an evaluation assignment participatory and self-reflective and thus an empowering experience for all involved. This document briefly describes the basic principles and elements of the process that I usually follow in evaluation assignments, in which the external evaluation is initiated by the funding agency as part of the existing funding contract.
First of all I confirm or negotiate with the funding agency that the ToR for the assignment allows for the process to be as participatory and self-reflective as possible. This includes organising workshops with the relevant staff/board to initiate and conclude the evaluation process. It also includes the review of the donor role. I prefer to de-link the evaluation

process from the funding decision moments, but this is often difficult to accomplish as most external evaluations are planned near the termination of a funding phase and are thus easily seen as an 'exam' that determines future (levels of) funding.

Step one: opening workshop
The task of the evaluators in the opening workshop with the staff of the NGO being evaluated is to get all agendas clearly on the table, review the ToR as it was drafted and make an inventory of different interests in and expectations about the evaluation. The listed expectations and interests need to be jointly analysed for their inclusion in the evaluation process. Time and scope limitations – and hence non-inclusion of certain expectations – need to be shared to avoid disappointments at the end.

It is also important to make an inventory of the fears and anxieties that staff and management (and board members) may have about the evaluation. Generally it takes a bit of probing – 'we have no fears about this evaluation' – before staff start sharing their often numerous anxieties, often including: 'we may lose our funding if mistakes are found', 'my job is at stake', 'the evaluators may have their biases', 'our board/management will not appreciate our sharing real facts', 'there will be too little time to capture all that has been done', 'the evaluators will not understand the difficult and unique situation we are working in'. These anxieties need to be carefully addressed as they may easily hamper an honest process of reflection. Specifically related to the sensitive issues of violence, sex and HIV and traditional cultural practices, both positive and harmful, there are often issues of both shame or pride that may easily cause anxieties: will the evaluation team consider these issues respectfully and within the context, can existing bad practices be shared without being instantly condemned?

The external evaluators need to present their 'credentials', who they are, whether or not they are independent of the funders or other direct stakeholders and what experiences and skills they bring to undertake the evaluation. It often helps to remove anxieties when I share that I too have been evaluated during programme implementation activities and that it can, indeed, be sensitive. Evaluators also need to share their views and principles regarding evaluations.

Based on my experience as consultant, frequently involved in external evaluations, I generally explain my role as that of a facilitator in a participatory evaluation process. I do not consider an evaluation to be an inspection or fault-finding exercise but rather a process of reflection, where the evaluation team functions as facilitators holding up a "transparent mirror" for the NGO to look back at the past performance, output and outcome, but also to look forward through the mirror, using the past knowledge and experiences as input. How do we view the past: what worked well and why, what did not work, and why? I always explain that it is as important to analyse what worked well and the elements (actions, people, leadership, contacts, cultural traditions) that contributed to that success as it is to acknowledge what weaknesses there have been, why these are weaknesses and who considers them to be weaknesses.

An exercise in this opening workshop to jointly analyse dreams that individual staff members have for the future (of the organisation and its work) and subsequently listing the elements that could turn the dreams into reality, both for programme and organisational matters, often brings out strengths and weaknesses in a much more positive tone than when focussing on weaknesses in a traditional SWOT analysis. A subsequent exercise where each staff member lists the five most important changes they would make to become more effective in the programme implemented and as organisation, if (s)he was in the director's position, concretises the SWOT to a very practical level: many of the proposed changes are common to the staff as a whole. This also sharpens issues to be further researched in the evaluation.

It helps to sharpen prioritising activities in situations where lots of new activities keep getting added to the programme of the NGO, to ask what should be stopped or kept if the NGO's budget would suddenly be reduced by 50%. What activities, campaigns, actions or services have had the greatest added value to the objectives the organisation wants to achieve: prevention of HIV infection and gender justice?
To bring the key issues to the table during this start-up process, an inventory (individual cards, plenary sharing) is made of what problems there are with respect to GBV and its inter-linkages with HIV, education and cultural practices, what could best be done in response to the problems analysed, what the NGO has concretely done and how that links to the earlier analysis of problems and responses, and – very importantly – whether the programme clientele (community groups, students, sex workers) would make the same analysis of problems, responses and what the NGO should do.

The evaluation can thus address what the NGO originally set out to do, and based on what analysis, what was/is really done (output) and subsequently what outcome and perhaps impact is expected and/or can be shown. The evaluation needs to establish who wanted the NGO to do what it has done. In other words: who did and does the NGO listen too? How does the NGO establish that what it does is useful, effective and the best way forward? What indicators does the NGO use for that? Ideally such indicators would already be in use, but many NGOs have not gone very far yet in developing indicators. Are the data that the NGO collects useful, does the NGO use case analysis, to what extent are attendance (training, rally, etc) numbers used and what do they indicate? The questioning helps to get the issues clear and commonly shared on the basis of which the evaluation can be conducted in a participatory way.

Step two: further planning the evaluation
Informed by the outcome of this workshop, a visit/interview schedule needs to be developed or an earlier plan refined and adapted if required. Whereas the evaluation team needs to maintain a level of independence in their choices, it is also important to engage the staff in listing the stakeholders whom they feel the evaluation team should meet to get an adequate picture: community groups, specific groups in the programme's clientele (including strong as well as weak examples), partners in campaigning, service providers, government officials (including police officials, members of the judiciary, school teachers) traditional leaders, religious leaders and perhaps politicians if they are being lobbied or supportive of the programme. This joint listing of stakeholders and partners may also indicate who the 'should be' stakeholders are, that have not been involved in the programme yet. In this participatory way, the evaluation process contributes to a maximum ownership of the assessment process by the organisation itself, also avoiding a later 'you have talked to the wrong people'. This

actually often serves to broaden ideas of who really does or should matter in the larger picture of what the organisation does.

Step three: 'fact' finding
This includes the interviews with staff and board, activity observation visits (e.g. training, workshops or campaigns), focus group discussions/individual interviews with relevant stakeholders/community groups etc. in areas of work, workshops, and surveys. Review of literature/documents, reports, publications. Time permitting and if feasible, site visits should be organised for comparison to communities/settings/villages not covered by the programme.

Step four: concluding workshop and sharing feedback on of findings' analysis
After all the interviews, focus group discussions or activity visits it is very important to organise a sharing, feedback and debriefing session with staff and (perhaps separately) board and whenever possible community groups/authorities/local leaders. This workshop at the end of the evaluation process will serve both to provide feedback based on the evaluation team findings and to share preliminary conclusions and recommendations, but also to check the validity and relevance of these conclusions and recommendations.

The more the staff and others consider the findings and its analysis as correct as well as the conclusions and recommendations, the more likely it will be that the organisation will take ownership of the evaluation process and its outcome and hence will undertake to implement the recommendations.

Rather than simply giving a debriefing presentation, including the teams' conclusions and recommendations, I generally present different elements separately and call for group discussions to review what was presented: first the programme/activities, second the organisation. During the group work feedback agreements and differences are discussed. The staff is subsequently asked to prepare their own conclusions and recommendations as they see fit based on agreed findings. This process has worked remarkably well to maximise ownership of the consequences of the findings presented and agreed. Only after the staff has presented and discussed their own conclusions and recommendations, the evaluation team shares what they had prepared before and subsequently the matches and differences are discussed. Given the transparent and continuously participatory process of collecting relevant facts and data, the matches between the conclusions and recommendations by the staff and those prepared by the evaluation team are generally very high.

What comes back quite often at the very end of such evaluation feedback workshops is that the appreciation for the jointly agreed conclusions and recommendations is mixed with anxiety as to whether the funding agencies, or even the NGO's own board, will understand and value this open acknowledgement of programmatic and institutional weaknesses and the ways the organisation wishes to address them, or whether it will be used to curtail funding, stop it altogether or introduce new conditions for its continuation. In response to that and based on my own experience I can share that the more organisations honestly share their problems and recognised weaknesses with serious donors as partners and indicate how they wish and concretely plan to address them, the more likely it will be that the donor is prepared to support the NGO in addressing these weaknesses as planned and may even provide additional support for that process, financially or otherwise. In the difficult and sensitive fields of abuse, violence, sexuality, sexual and reproductive health, gender justice and HIV prevention there are many hurdles to be overcome in relation to power and patriarchy. There are cultural traditions and norms to be addressed, both within organisations (including staff members' own norms, values and experiences of abuse) and in the campaigns and services provided. Such problems and weaknesses are not to be ignored or denied but need to be addressed. Of course funding agencies have a right to demand from their partners to bring in basic programmatic qualities and institutional capacities at the time of negotiating the partnership. But they also have a duty to support NGOs in further capacity development. NGOs also need to be transparent and firm about their own strengths and weaknesses: funding agencies, who expect their partners to be perfect institutions with only successful programmes that can be shown to the back-donors at home, can best be ignored as partner: "they obviously don't understand what development is all about".

Step five: report drafting, feedback and follow-up by funding agency and recipient NGO
After a draft version of the evaluation report, feedback by the NGO and the funding agency in terms of clarity or factual errors, a final version of the evaluation report is sent to both contracting parties. The follow-up to an evaluation process includes formulating responses by the NGO and the funding agency with respect to the recommendations made, with specific attention to strengthening the capacity to meaningfully monitor and evaluate the very process of change they are engaged in.

References
Imam, Ayesha, Simon Matsvai and Jan Reynders. "Evaluating Social Change Networks: Women in Law and Development in Africa" In: *Measuring the Immeasurable, Planning, Monitoring and Evaluation of Networks*. Marilee Karl (ed.) New Delhi, India: Women's Feature Service/Novib, 1998.

About the authors

Eliezer F. Wangulu
Eliezer F. Wangulu is a writer and editor specialised in population and health communication. He holds an MA degree in journalism studies from Cardiff University, Wales, United Kingdom. He has 20 years of professional experience accumulated in Kenya, The Netherlands, Somaliland, South Africa and Zimbabwe. Wangulu has edited publications, undertaken media training and managed media projects. He has been head researcher in the production of several documentaries and undertaken media consultancies for national and international organisations. He is currently Managing Editor of *Exchange on HIV and AIDS, Sexuality and Gender* magazine at the Royal Tropical Institute (KIT) in Amsterdam, The Netherlands.

Contact: e.wangulu@kit.nl

Lois Barbara Chingandu
Lois Chingandu is the Executive Director of Southern Africa HIV and AIDS Information Dissemination Service (SAfAIDS). She has over 15 years' experience in designing and managing HIV and AIDS and health programmes in Africa. She has an in-depth understanding of HIV and AIDS prevention, treatment, care, gender, orphans and vulnerable children (OVC) issues acquired during her work with marginalised communities in southern Africa.
Lois has used this experience at SAfAIDS to develop and publish a variety of HIV and AIDS materials including books and toolkits for mobilising and training service providers and communities on various HIV and AIDS-related issues. She has played a critical role in advocating policy changes for the betterment of women and children in southern Africa and beyond.
Lois was responsible for conceptualising and designing the innovative 'Changing the River's Flow Programme' that addresses cultural norms, values and structures that fuel the HIV epidemic in Africa.

Contact: lois@safaids.net

Ngoni Chibukire
Ngoni is an Economist by profession and holds an MSc in Economics from the University of Zimbabwe. He has over nine years' experience in research and health economics, with specific focus on the economics of the HIV and AIDS epidemic. Ngoni is currently SAfAIDS' Regional Head for Capacity Development. His unit is responsible for all capacity development-related activities in 10 southern Africa countries where the regional NGO operates. He has six years of experience in establishment and evaluation of HIV and AIDS programmes and policies in the World of Work for NGOs across the southern African region.

Contact: Ngoni@safaids.net

Virginia Maserame Mojapele
Maserame is a nurse and community health specialist by profession. She holds a Masters Degree in Community Health Nursing from the Medical University of Limpopo, South Africa. She is currently the Programme Manager with SAfAIDS. Maserame has worked in the field of health and development for private and public sectors in southern Africa for 10 years. She has also worked for South Africa's Ministry of Health at national, provincial and district levels before joining the NGO sector where she has been working in the areas of public health, HIV and AIDS and gender both at regional and international levels. Her areas of interest include community needs assessments, programme implementation, policy and guidelines development, programme and business plan development, implementation, evaluation, culture, gender based-violence and women's rights trainings. Maserame also mentors and coaches health and development professionals.

Contact: Maserame@safaids.net

Anke van der Kwaak
Anke van der Kwaak holds a Master of Science degree in Cultural Anthropology with specialisation in gender and health, health systems research, and culture and health. She has several years' experience as a researcher and trainer in these fields in Africa and Asia. Anke has worked for 10 years as a university lecturer at the Medical Faculty of the Vrije Universteit (Free University) in Amsterdam, The Netherlands. She is a senior advisor and researcher in sexuality, sexual health, capacity development in research and quality of care.

Contact: a.v.d.kwaak@kit.nl

Francis Obare, PhD
Francis Obare is a Demographer and holds a PhD degree from the University of Pennsylvania in the United States. He has nine years' experience in research in the areas of health and mortality with specific focus on inequalities in access to maternal and child health services, adolescent health, sexual and reproductive health, and HIV and AIDS. His research spans a number of countries in eastern and southern Africa including Ethiopia, Kenya, Malawi and Uganda. Francis is currently a Senior Analyst with the Population Council in Nairobi, Kenya.

Contact: obareonyango@yahoo.com

Hermen Ormel
Hermen Ormel is a social anthropologist with a postgraduate degree in Public Health (MPH). He works with the Netherlands' Royal Tropical Institute (KIT) as Senior Advisor, mainly on sexual and reproductive health and rights and HIV and AIDS issues. Hermen has worked on capacity development for research, gender issues, young people and local responses for HIV in Africa, Asia and Latin America.
Contact: h.ormel@kit.nl

Olloriak Sawade
Olloriak Sawade is the Policy Advisor on education in the Research and Development Bureau at Oxfam Novib. She worked in Canada, Ghana and Thailand on issues around

education, child's rights, health and the environment before joining Oxfam Novib (ON). Olloriak did her masters degree at the University of Amsterdam and her research thesis focused on education and fragile states.

Contact: olloriak.sawade@oxfamnovib.nl

Jeanette Kloosterman, PhD
Jeanette Kloosterman works as Policy Advisor at the Research and Development department at Oxfam Novib on The Right to an Identity: Gender and Diversity. Before joining the organisation, she worked for almost 10 years in the global South, first with the United Nation's Food and Agriculture Organisation (FAO)-VN and then with the European Union (EU) in different rural development projects on social forestry and gender equality in indigenous contexts (LA). Her PhD research at the University of Utrecht (Netherlands) was about identity and collective rights of indigenous peoples.

Contact: jeanette.kloosterman@oxfamnovib.nl

Josephine Pedun
Josephine Pedun is a Programme Officer at Forum for African Women Educationalists (FAWE) Uganda Chapter. She previously worked with Uganda's Ministry of Gender, Labour and Social Development. Pedun has also worked for several years in the area of gender, child rights and policy. She holds an MA Degree in Social Sector Planning and Management, which she obtained from Makerere University, Kampala, Uganda.

Contact: jpedun2005@yahoo.com

Rashida Parveen
Rashida Parveen is the Programme Manager, Adolescent Development Programme, BRAC in Bangladesh. She has been with BRAC for more than 20 years. Parveen is responsible for developing strategies and policies for adolescent development and ensuring BRAC's smooth liaison with other organisations. She has also been active in planning and designing the BRAC Education Programme and has published many books for children, teachers and adolescents. Parveen undertook her Postgraduate studies in Human Resources Development from Niagara College in Ontario, Canada. She also holds an MA Degree from the Rajshahi University in Bangladesh.

Contact: rashida.p@brac.net

Cheikhou Toure
Cheikhou Touré is a consultant on quality education and he is an education specialist at Enda Graf Sahel in Senegal. He has been a primary and secondary teacher and a university lecturer. Toure has also been a school inspector and was a director in the Ministry of Education in Senegal.

Contact: toure_cheikhou@yahoo.fr

Ndéye Adama Carine Mbengue
Ndéye Adama Carine Mbengue is currently Programme Manager at FAWE Senegal chapter. She has a Masters in Business Administration and a diploma in Development Programmes. Adama has worked for 10 years in the education sector specifically focusing on gender equity for girls and women.

Jan Reynders
Jan Reynders holds an MA degree in Development Studies. He has worked in the field of international development cooperation for over 35 years, both hands-on in the field (in Bangladesh) and as manager and policy advisor in a Dutch funding agency. Since 1994, Reynders has been an independent gender-justice and development consultant and he has undertaken assignments in over 30 countries in Africa, Asia, the Caribbean and (central and eastern) Europe for international, national and local NGOs, international social change networks, international funding agencies, donor governments, technical assistance agencies, UN agencies and academic institutions.
He serves on the board of the Gender and Water Alliance (GWA) and the board of the Dutch Gender Platform (WO=MEN). Reynders is active in its men's working group 'The Kitchen Table' which is a member of MenEngage.

Contact: Reynders.Jan@net.HCC.nl

Colophon

Royal Tropical Institute (KIT)
KIT Information & Library Services
PO Box 95001
1090 HA Amsterdam
The Netherlands
E: ILS@kit.nl
W: www.kit.nl

KIT Publishers
PO Box 95001
1090 HA Amsterdam
The Netherlands
E: publishers@kit.nl
W: www.kitpublishers.nl

© 2011 – KIT Publishers, Amsterdam

Graphic design: Grafisch Ontwerpbureau Agaatsz bNO, Meppel
Cover design: Natalie Davies, SAfAIDS
Printing: Bariet, Ruinen

The publication of this book was funded by KIT.

ISBN 978 94 6022 1415